I0103882

LIVING WITH A KNEE REPLACEMENT
BEND IT; USE IT; ENJOY IT

Available from www.lulu.com

LIVING WITH A KNEE REPLACEMENT
BEND IT; USE IT; ENJOY IT

by

David P. Mellinger

The contents are a description of the experience of recovery from men and women who have had knee replacement surgery.

First House on the Block
Kearney, Nebraska

© 2010 by David P. Mellinger

ISBN 978-0-615-39577-7

Publisher: First House on the Block
        4003 Bel Air Dr.
        Kearney, NE 68845
        Email: kneebone.mellinger@gmail.com

Acknowledgements

To those who talk of miracles, I acknowledge that having new knees is a great blessing. I thank my dear wife, Paula, for sticking with me, not only through our forty-three years together, but also the years of suffering before the surgeries and the recovery after. The blessing of new knees would not have been possible without the skill of Dr. Mark Meyer, my surgeon, and Joel McReynolds his Physician's Assistant at Kearney Bone & Joint Clinic in Kearney Nebraska.

I also want to thank those who directly contributed their stories; Joel McReynolds, PA-C, MPAS, Scott Arens, ATC, Gisele, Barb, Mike, Roxann, Vicki, Bennie, Joanna, and others not mentioned by name.

Contents

INTRODUCTION

The idea for this book grew out of a conversation with Gisele, another recovering total knee recipient in the physical therapy gym. She was forty-seven, I was sixty-three. We began talking about what we had experienced after leaving the hospital and realized no one in the doctor's office, the hospital, or the physical therapy office had said anything about what to expect after leaving the hospital. The doctors and hospital briefed us fully about how to prepare for the surgery, but there was little guidance on what would happen when we woke up. There was precious little information, beyond medicines to take, on what we would experience when we went home. And we learned nothing about what to expect during recovery.

The care we received in the hospital was simply wonderful. All the doctors and nurses did their jobs in a caring and professional manner. We left with good memories of having been well cared for. Then the lights went off.

10

The hospital discharged us with our prescriptions for pain killers, stool softeners and blood thinners. We had a walker or crutch to get around. We had an ice pack. We had a list of exercises to do (The same list as when we went into the hospital.) We had the warning to get prophylactic antibiotics when we had dental work or our teeth cleaned.

When we left the hospital we had instructions on how to get into the car – a complicated process when your knee does not bend and hurts every time you think about moving it. The nurse's aide who pushed the wheelchair to the curb waved goodbye. From that point on it was like falling into a black hole. The actual experience of being home was a lot more complicated than we had expected.

Gisele and I, as we talked in the gym during physical therapy, realized that both of us were reaching the same milestones of recovery and were doing it in about the same length of time, in spite of the sixteen year difference in our ages. This short book will help the reader anticipate the steps to expect in recovery and when to expect them. Knowing what is coming makes the next steps easier to deal with, and attending to what steps already achieved brings hope for success at each step.

Men and women who have gone through the process of healing and know from experience what is involved in recovery from knee replacement surgery wrote this book. Doctors and medical professionals did have input during the writing.

Before I had my first operation I did not think much about who has knee replacements. All I knew is that my knee hurt and I wanted the pain to stop. I did later ask Joel McReynolds, who works as a Physician's Assistant for the surgeon who did my knees, about who has knees replaced. The age ranges from teens, after bone growth has stopped, all the way to people in their nineties. Cancer might trigger the need for a total replacement in a teenager. For the rest of us pain was enough motivation to go ahead and agree to surgery. Joel says, "The decision for surgery is based on the pain and dysfunction, with medical evaluation to determine the ability of the patient to successfully recover from the procedure." In Joel's experience the age group from sixty to eighty is a "common age range for total knee arthroplasty. However, the lower and upper age limits both seem to be widening in the last decade."

That means you are probably between sixty and eighty if you have had your knee replaced and there is a two out of three chance that you are going home to recover. Joel adds, "The determining factors to return home depend on the patient's pre-arthroplasty functional level, their motivation, and the support system for home needs."

If you are reading this book before your surgery, here are some things you can do to make it easier when you go home. The most important step is to work at getting strength in the leg which is going to get the new knee. If you are like I was, you have limped through the pain in your knee for years and have done as little physical activity as possible. In the gym, Gisele talked about having to think about how far she would have to walk when she went shopping, and I talked about how much my old knee hurt each day, starting with my morning walk to the bathroom.

The muscles in your leg may be weak from not using them, and the surgery itself can weaken them even more. Your surgeon, or the hospital when you go in for your pre-op orientation, will give you a sheet of instructions on exercises to do before entering the hospital for your surgery. The exercises work directly on the muscles which the operation affects. The stronger your muscles are when you go in for surgery, the faster you will heal when you go home.

When you get home from the hospital, you will need a place to sit where you can put your leg up. Take my word for it; you will not be able to sit comfortably in a regular chair for some time. After my first surgery I moved a recliner next to my bed. By the time I had my other knee replacement I felt comfortable having the recliner in an adjoining room. I was able to hobble between the chair, the bathroom, and my bed.

It is also a good idea to have a TV close by. The knee recipients I talked to had a hard time concentrating enough to read until some time after the surgery. Like them, I watched a lot of daytime television between naps. You will find yourself sleeping a lot during the first few weeks; though sleeping through the night is more challenging.

And you will need to think about how to meet nature's call. Most people do not realize that a standard toilet seat is much lower than a normal chair. I found this out only after getting out of the hospital. If you do not have something solid, the edge of a counter, a firmly attached handicap bar or a willing helper, to lever yourself down and up, you can get a booster seat to temporarily put on your toilet to make it easier to get on and off. One knee recipient said she got a bad bruise from using a booster seat. I was discreet enough not to inquire about the exact nature of the bruising.

I also bought an inexpensive plastic stool with adjustable legs for the bathtub. It was a treat to be able to sit and let the shower run over me without worrying about whether I was going to fall over.

The Senior Center in our city has a roomful of walkers, canes, crutches, risers, etc, which one can rent for about $10.00.

Throughout the book you will read about "tricks." Tricks are simply the things you will be able to do as the swelling goes out of the knee and recovery progresses. Thinking of each new step taken as a trick is one way of celebrating progress. Celebrating a small gain helps to make the wait between big steps easier.

There is an old joke about a man who had his fingers crushed in an accident. While the doctor was patching him up the man asked, "Doc, will I be able to play the piano?"

The doctor replied, "Sure, your hand will be just fine."

The man answered with a grin, "Great, I never could play the piano before."

The moral of the story is that a knee replacement may not let you do things you could not do before your original joint wore out.

The good news is that the knee recipients I talked to were mostly able to resume the activities they had to give up because of the pain from their worn out knee joint. I have had my knees for over a year. People still ask, "Does it still hurt?" Their second question is, "Is it as good as new?" The answer to the first question is a qualified, "No." After twelve months the "Uni" or partial knee replacement still has twinges that I occasionally need to walk off. At eighteen months, the total replacement does not give me any pain.

The answer to the second question is, "No, it's not as good as the original equipment when it was new, but it's a lot better than the worn out knee before the operation". There really are some restrictions on what the prosthetic knee will tolerate. Each recipient will have a somewhat different list of things they can and cannot do with the new knee. In general, replacement knees are great for walking and climbing stairs. They are not good for running or for heavy lifting. How long will any particular knee replacement last? Most doctors say about twenty years. Not bad.

Vicki told me her doctor stressed to her, "Just remember your knee will never be normal." The doctor's warning was dire; however, Vicki says she now, after nine months, sometimes forgets she has a new knee.

I want to stress that recovery from knee surgery is an active process. A common perception about having an operation is that we go into surgery and the doctor "fixes" what is wrong. All we have to do afterward is rest up for as long as the doctor says. With knee replacement surgery, the operation does fix the joint, but it is up to the patient to actively recover. Actively recovering takes a lot of time and effort.

Unfortunately, recovery from knee replacement surgery is not like a TV show or a movie in which the hero solves every problem in an hour – less commercial time. It is more like a whole seasons worth of stories, on a show that does resolve the issues at the end of the year. Too many shows leave you hanging at the end of the season.

This book targets those knee recipients who anticipate going home from the hospital. It assumes you are one of those knee recipients who plan on getting back to being active. Not all knee recipients fit that description. About one in three will go first to a care facility for rehabilitation, either because of medical conditions or because there is no one at home to help them in those first few critical weeks. If you are thinking about going home and there is no one available to help, I encourage you to look into a short term stay at a care facility.

To make the story of recovery more organized, most of the narrative is based on my experience, that of a relatively in shape sixty-three year old man. The frequent use of "I" in the manuscript is uncomfortable for the writer since the intent is not to focus on me but to show the pace of recovery and give examples of the range of experiences of knee recipients in recovery. The stories and experiences of other knee recipients are liberally included to show the range of what we have gone through.

This book is on recovery, not problems. Problems are mentioned only in passing as they interfere with recovery. If you have problems during your recovery, please consult your doctor.

I hope your experience of healing from knee replacement surgery goes smoothly, and leads to full recovery.

PART ONE

RECOVERY STARTS IN THE HOSPITAL

(The first week)

Each of us who has an artificial knee, either "Total" or "Uni" (a replacement of only half of the knee) has gone through a stay in the hospital. There are differences in our experiences based on where the operation occurred, age, health, and/or level of functioning before surgery. In spite of these differences, much of the experience is similar. I had my surgeries at Good Samaritan Hospital in Kearney, Nebraska where the usual hospital experience is to go in early on a Monday for the surgery with discharge on Thursday if there are no complications. I was fortunate to be able to follow that pattern for both the total right knee replacement in April of 2007 and the partial left knee in October of 2007.

ONE

MONDAY: The Day of the Big Cut

There are several steps which typically lead up to the big day. The first step is just realizing that the pain from your deteriorating knee is interfering with your life. Many people who decide to have a knee replaced have endured the pain for years. I found myself limping heavily for about five years. I could not walk a block without resting. I curtailed many activities such as being a tourist, walking with my wife, working with Habitat For Humanity, mowing the lawn (I am blessed with a wife who does not mind mowing), and almost anything that involved walking or being on my feet for any length of time.

Each night I was exhausted from simply trying to get to work, get home and do the minimum of chores at home. I was not unique in that experience. Each of the knee recipients I talked to had a similar experience. Some had endured years of treatment, injections, etc. trying to nurse the knee along until their doctor told them they were old enough to have the joint replaced.

The end result is that the potential knee recipient often reluctantly makes an appointment with their doctor to discuss the pain and the possibility of having a knee replaced.

Mike said the story began for him in April with a "simple" arthroscopic surgery (in arthroscopic surgery the doctor makes a few small slits in the skin and inserts the tools through them; full recovery takes about two weeks.) "The simple part disappeared when the surgeon could find no meniscus (cartilage that acts as a shock absorber in the joint) to work with. I decided to have micro-surgery; punching holes in the bone to make it bleed to form scar tissue as a cushion between the bones. After nine weeks on crutches, off my left leg, it was determined the surgery failed. I made a decision to have a total knee replacement."

My own decision was quicker and made when I visited my family doctor. He knew me well from shared activities in our church and the community. When I finally made the appointment, I went in and said, "It's time to talk about my knee."

The doctor looked me in the eye and said, "I've seen you walk. It's time to do something." He turned to his prescription pad and wrote a referral to an orthopedic surgeon. My doctor ordered blood tests and x-rays to determine if I was well enough for surgery

The only choice I got to make was which surgeon was going to do the operation. That was all it took.

Sometime after the results of all the tests came back, I had a consultation with the surgeon. He was the same surgeon who rebuilt my knee twenty-five years ago when I wore it out from road racing. *That is another whole story.*

A week before the big day, I had an appointment at the hospital to fill out a long pre-operation questionnaire about medical conditions, current medications, insurance and all the other details that need to be taken care of before surgery. The admissions clerk told me to, "Come to the hospital at six in the morning on the day of surgery. Oh, and don't eat or drink after midnight."

The day inevitably came. Six in the morning is early. Maybe they wanted me to be there before I woke up enough to chicken out. I certainly had told myself many times before this day that the knee was not so bad. So it started hurting by the time I got from my bed to the bathroom in the morning. It wasn't that bad! I found myself sitting in a cold waiting room with my wife, Paula, who was not going to let me back out, and trying to avoid eye contact with the other nervous people waiting for the same fate as I was facing.

The nurses and helpers were very sympathetic through all the preparations. At the appointed time, I was taken into the pre-operation preparation room. The room was divided into little compartments by drawn curtains. Each compartment was just large enough for a bed, a chair, and an equipment stand. I really didn't see anyone else. It was as if each of us who were heading for an operating room disappeared as they entered.

The nurse told me to go into a small room, much like a department store changing room and dress in the fashionable open backed gown that hospitals use and get into bed. I undressed and held the back of my robe closed while I crossed the room to disappear into my cubicle.

Once in bed, the nurse hooked me up to an intravenous drip and covered me with a warm blanket. Those warm blankets are nice. They even gave one to my wife as she waited by my side. At least three times, a nurse or doctor asked me to point to the site of the operation. Before the preparations for surgery were finished, my knee bore my autograph and those of the surgeon, physician's assistant, and at least one nurse. I did appreciate the efforts to make sure they worked on the right spot.

The nurse put some kind of medication through the IV into my arm. For the first operation on my right knee, that's the last thing I remember. By the second operation on my left knee, I was awake all the way to the operating room. When I asked why I remembered so much the second time, they told me that some people are more nervous and get more happy meds. I must have been pretty nervous the first time.

Everything after that is a blank.

Some people have more memory of the day they have surgery than others. I simply did not remember anything until I woke up in the hospital bed Tuesday morning. All I have is stories from my wife telling people what goofy things I said. She says one time I opened my eyes and said, "This is a very good steak I'm having," and then drifted off again. That was an odd thing for me to say, since I got sick on the gelatin and crackers at suppertime.

I don't even remember Paula being there when I woke up from the anesthetic. I wasn't surprised. My usual response to being sick is to pull the covers over my head and not come out until I feel better. Having no memory for the day of the surgery is not all bad. I have a feeling it was not a day I would want to remember.

TWO

TUESDAY: Waking Up for Real

One patient who has had numerous joint replacements due to rheumatoid arthritis said, "Recovery begins when you wake up screaming." In a way, that is a pretty good description of waking up on the day after surgery. The anesthesia has worn off, the pain has set in, and the nurse has not come in with a pain pill, or, if you have a Patient Controlled Analgesia button, you've forgotten how to use it.

You will likely wake up earlier than you expected or wanted. Someone from the lab will come in around 5:00 AM for blood work. They come in early so, if the lab results show any problem, your doctor will know of any issues before he or she does rounds. A nurse comes in to take your vital signs for the same reason. Someone from the physical therapy department comes in to adjust the knobs on any apparatus which is hanging over your bed. The apparatus is to help the patient position his or her self if they need something to grab on to while moving around in the bed. I never did figure out why the physical therapy people came in so early to tighten knobs.

When I finally woke up that first day, there was an IV needle stuck in my hand. I later remembered that the nurse had inserted the line before surgery. The IV is used for glucose solution, pain medications, antibiotics, and other things the doctor orders pumped into you. The needle did not hurt and did not get in the way, though this differs from patient to patient. One person I talked to said that she has veins which are hard to find and did not easily accept needles. She said she had quite a bit of pain from the IV. From what I understand, any pain or bruising from the needle will not cause permanent damage.

I also had an oxygen cannula in my nose. A cannula is any tube stuck into the body to drain fluids or administer medications. The cannula delivers oxygen to the patient following surgery. I had trouble keeping my oxygen up to the proper level. It seemed like every time I rolled over I cut off the oxygen flow and set off the alarm on the oxygen machine next to the bed. The alarm was an annoying high pitched beep, which brought the nurse to push a button and make sure there was no real problem. I felt like I was constantly apologizing for setting off the alarm when I felt fine and had no trouble breathing. Not everyone remembers having oxygen the following day.

You will wake up lying on your back. You will probably just need to get used to this position. It may be the only way that you can lay for a while. Pain, swelling, and a knee that will not bend make it impossible for one to do more than shift his or her buns a little to get some relief. I have talked to some knee recipients who were able to lie on their side with a pillow between their legs, but I could not lie on my side until long after I was out of the hospital.

There is a bulge underneath the blanket where your knee used to be. The topmost layer of this bulge is an ice pack, which will be a constant companion. Underneath the ice pack are the operated knee and its dressing. The top layer of the dressing is a gauze wrap. Beneath the gauze the operated knee is swathed in a big fat wad of cotton batting to absorb any minimal blood seepage from the incision. Under the cotton batting are metal staples every quarter to half inch. The staples hold the incision together like old fashioned stitches until the skin has a chance to heal. A dermatologist told me the stainless steel staples are faster to put in and are less likely to pull out on a big incision.

Beneath all those layers is a lot of swelling. The new joint itself is perfectly fine. The cement used to attach the prosthetic appliance to the bones had set completely a few minutes after your surgeon installed the joint, and the new knee is quite stable by the time you wake up. While you were safely asleep in the operating room, your surgeon flexed and straightened the joint as far as it would go, to be certain it worked properly. Joel, my surgeon's Physician's Assistant said that the joint would bend about 105 degrees right after surgery. There is no need to worry about harming the joint by moving it. Though moving the knee does hurt – a lot!

The pain is not overwhelming when you first wake up, but it increases as the surgical anesthetic wears off during the day and you become more alert. When the knee starts to hurt more than you think you can stand, you may have what my hospital called a Patient Controlled Analgesic device. The PAC has a magic button which connects to the IV. You can push the button and get a dose of powerful narcotic pain killer. You need not be concerned about overdosing. The button is set so an overdose is impossible. With the PAC the patient is partly in control of how much medicine he or she receives. Most people actually use less medication than if they have to call a nurse for a shot or a pill. Also do not be concerned by the word narcotic. What you are taking is a medicine and not a "drug" that you will get hooked on.

One woman reacted to the narcotic pain killer by becoming nauseous. If you have nausea and it gets too bad, you can ask the nurse for an anti-nausea medicine. The good news about being sick to your stomach from meds or an anesthesia hangover is that vomiting usually does not make the knee hurt.

I had a urinal to use when needed. It sounds gross, but having some risk of a bedpan spill is better than trying to get out of bed and walk all the way across the room. I did have a bedpan spill in the middle of the night. While I was a bit embarrassed, I finally decided that the only thing I could do was push the call button. The night nurse, thankfully a male, smiled and helped me get cleaned up as if cleaning up after patients was something he did every day.

At this point you still have not been out of bed, much less tried to walk. I did not even try to get out of bed to go to the bathroom for several days. If I was already up, I would head in the direction of the bathroom, but I wasn't going to make a special trip. Because of the surgery and not eating since Sunday night, I did not have a bowel movement for several days. I counted that as a small blessing.

My situation, with regard to getting out of bed, was better than Roxann's. She had her surgery in a hospital in another town. "I had both knees replaced on August 4, 2008. I went from the surgery suite to joint camp. While I was there I was gotten up the first night to go to the bathroom after being handed my walker and assisted with my gripper socks. Good Lord, the bathroom was waaay over there and you expect me to walk over there???? Yup, in no uncertain terms. You need to go, you need to walk. I was surprised at what little pain I did have but the night was young, and with fluids running I needed to go again and again."

Unfortunately, some people react to the anesthesia and throw up everything they eat. I had a horrible time with nausea. I could not keep anything down until the evening and that was just crackers and some juice. In spite of the reputation of hospital food for being less than tasty, I was thankful when I was finally able to keep some food down.

I also noticed an uncomfortable pressure on my feet. My feet felt like something was squeezing them. After about ten seconds, I heard a hiss and the pressure on my feet released. Then the squeezing started again. This went on and on and on; pressure, release, pressure, release. I finally asked the nurse what was going on. She pulled back the covers. Little booties encased my feet. The booties were attached to hoses that ran down to the floor and a machine of some kind.

The official name of the booties is Pneumatic Foot Pump device. They do have a purpose beyond acting like a sort of Chinese water torture – drip, drip, drip – which may cause a response from the patient in the nature of, "I can't take it anymore. Make it stop." At least that was my response. My nurses, kind as they were, did not heed my plea.

The booties promote circulation and prevent blood clots while the patient spends so much time in bed. The booties were less uncomfortable when I had the nurse remove the hospital-issue, light tan, non-slip socks whenever she strapped on the booties. Either way, the constant squeeze and release was the most uncomfortable part of being in the hospital. After I had been out of bed the first time, the relief from the squeezing was a strong motivator to get out of bed again and have the booties off for a while.

Breakfast was no thrill for me. I was still throwing up. But if you don't have that problem you will get to start on solid food the day following surgery. The first day's food will depend on how you are doing coming out of the anesthesia. I was limited to liquids and gelatin, with maybe some crackers, none of which I could keep down. The nausea was still with me. If you fare better than I, you might be able to eat a meal, though the meals are light at first. It takes some time for the bowels to get started again after surgery and the light food helps.

Also on the day after surgery, you will have a chance to wash up while in bed. The nurse brings in a wash pan filled with warm water, a washrag, and a towel. Even though you are still in bed and feeling pretty wretched, it's nice to have some warm water and soap on your face. You also get to brush your teeth. These two activities help you feel a little bit normal.

Sometime after you have cleaned up, a nurse comes in to change the dressing on your knee. When all the wrapping is off, and if everything is going well with your knee, you will be surprised at how little blood is present. It will be your first chance to see the incision, which isn't pretty. There is a long ugly cut, about six inches long, pulled together every quarter inch or so by steel staples. The incision runs right along the front of the knee from several inches above to several inches below. There are puckers of skin sticking up here and there along the incision, like mismatched patches of land along an earthquake fault. The incision for a partial knee replacement is a bit shorter, but just as ugly.

The knee will be grossly swollen, maybe twice its normal size. The first impression of many who have replacement knees is something like, "What have they done to me?" Of course you always have the option of not looking at the incision, though you will have to look at it eventually. One benefit of taking a look now is that the first shock will be over with. Some of us were curious enough that we wanted to rush in and gawk.

If all is well, the incision is not bleeding beyond, perhaps, a little seepage. The staples actually do a wonderful job of holding the skin together. There will be bruising around the knee. After all, the surgeon sliced through the skin, pulled the joint out of the opening, sawed off chunks of bone, drilled holes into the long bones, pounded the prosthesis in place, bent the knee, stuffed it all

31

back into place, and then stapled the skin together. The bruising is a normal part of the operation and will eventually fade. How much of a scar remains, depends upon how you heal. Some of us scar worse than others.

The new dressing is much smaller. The nurse overlaps four-inch gauze pads down the length of the incision and holds them in place with a tube of elastic material that reaches from mid calf to mid thigh. The material they used on me was very much like the material in an elastic bandage. The new dressing is not at all bulky. The nurse changes the dressing each day.

One knee recipient said her doctor prescribed support hose to reduce swelling in her legs and feet. Roxann spoke of her long, sexy, white stockings. That's a good way to put a positive spin on the subject. A third woman said she had to wear the long hose for several weeks except when she was in bed. Fortunately, I never had to go that route.

Shortly after the nurse changed the dressing a therapist from physical therapy arrived to get me up for the first time. I don't recall if I the nurses warned me that the physical therapy folks were coming. I do remember my reaction to the idea of getting out of bed was along the lines of, "No way! I'm staying right where I am."

In spite of my resistance to the idea, I laid a smile over my grimace and did what they told me, which was to get out of bed. The first step in getting out of bed is to scoot your body to the edge of the mattress. Yes, it hurts to move. If the operated leg is on the near side, a helper will first support your foot and lift the operated leg over the edge of the bed. If the operated leg is on the far side, you can swing the good leg over the edge first then the helper lifts the operated leg off the edge of the bed and sets it gently on the floor.

I prayed that whoever was holding the operated leg did not drop it. No one did. After lying in bed for most of two days, I was a bit dizzy setting up for the first time and appreciated having someone there to help keep me steady. The process of getting out of bed is cumbersome if only one knee is replaced. With two new knees, it is harder yet. I spoke to one double knee patient who, when asked how they managed to get out of bed, simply responded, "Very carefully."

Standing is a scary thing. There is a natural tendency to resist putting pressure on bones that the surgeon has so recently carved up in order to install the new parts. The first time you stand, remember that the cement used to connect the parts of the new knee to your bones is completely set and the doctor has bent the knee to its full extent while in the operating room. Even so, it is scary to put weight on the joint for the first time. Standing does hurt a lot, but the pain is bearable. Though it does hurt to stand on the operated leg, all the pain is from when the surgeon reduced the bone for the new knee joint and from soft tissue swelling. Putting weight on the appliance does not add to the pain or do any injury. Your steps will be halting and slow, but do try to put your weight on the operated leg with each step and not hop on the good leg. Sharing weight on both legs will pay off with a faster recovery.

The physical therapists brought a walker for me to use for support. They also brought what the therapist called a "gait belt." The gait belt is a long web belt that buckles around the patient's waist. The helper holds onto the belt for additional support. How long the belt is used depends on how secure the patient appears to the therapist.

One "double knee" had crutches from the beginning. Most of the people I talked to used a walker rather than crutches to steady themselves.

Learning to use a walker is a trick of its own. Unfortunately, no one taught me how to do this trick. At first, I wanted to stand behind the rear legs of the walker and lean forward on it. Standing behind the walker made me put my weight on the handles and support myself on my arms. Leaning forward is awkward and tiring. This was probably a way of keeping some of the weight off my knee in order to assuage my lingering fear that my new knee would break if I put my full weight on it.

The four legged walker helps the user keep their balance, not support the user's weight. The device works best for balance when the user steps forward into the box formed by the legs of the walker. Standing in the box lets the user stand upright and have his or her legs support their weight. Standing in the box also is more stable with less risk of falling. Don't hesitate to tell the physical therapy staff if your walker seems to be too high or too low for comfort. A properly fitted walker will leave your arms just about straight when you use it.

One recipient said she had a walker with wheels on the front legs and it was easy for her to push when she walked. A walker with wheels sounds like a good thing to ask for.

Once I was standing, the gait belt around my waist and my hands clutching the grips of the walker, the physical therapist told me to walk to the door of my room and back. That door looked to be about a mile and a half away. The therapist hovered at my side while I baby-stepped over to the door and back. I may have whined that it hurt too much, but that did no good. Once you have walked on the new knee a few times you find that the pain is manageable and that walking gets easier.

That was enough. I went back to bed, secretly proud that I had not fallen on my face.

The therapists said "We'll be back this afternoon to take you to the gym."

I wasn't amused.

After you have had help getting out of bed the first time, the question arises whether you should do it yourself. My strategy was to try to do everything I could by myself as soon as I could. After all, I was going to have to go home in a few days and wanted to be sure I could make it out of bed. The next time the physical therapists came in, I asked them to stand by while I tried to get out of bed on my own. The physical therapists seemed pleased that I was trying to do things myself and were gracious enough to teach me a couple of self-help tricks.

The first trick I needed to learn was how to get the operated leg off the bed. The quadriceps muscle of the operated leg is still too weak to lift the leg on its own, or to support the leg below the knee. I wouldn't be able to get into or out of bed until I was able to lift up my operated leg. The trick is to hook the foot from the good leg under the heel of the operated leg and lift it onto or off the bed, or lift

35

it up to get the foot rest of a lounge chair raised. This is a good trick to get in and out of resting places without help. It is also a trick that the knee recipient needs to abandon as soon as their operated leg is strong enough to do the work itself.

After being out of bed for the first time you will be encouraged to spend time sitting up. My hospital room had a lounge chair I could sit in when I was not in bed. A lounge chair is nice since you can both lift the leg and lean back to rest. Sitting helps the lungs work more naturally, and reduces risk of pneumonia. Sitting up is also good practice for when the physical therapist takes you to the gym and the work is harder. After I had been on my back for most of two days, sitting up was also just plain enjoyable. An hour at a time that first day might be as much as you can handle without the pain getting to be too great. It was certainly enough for me. Every day the sitting up time got longer, though it was several weeks before sitting up time was longer than "on my back" time.

The second trick the therapist taught me was how to sit down. It is natural to back up to a chair with both feet a few inches out from the seat and sit down, bending the knees equally. This approach does not work when the operated knee does not flex beyond a few degrees. Sitting on a chair takes more than ninety degrees of flexibility in the knee and you do not have that right now. The doctor bent your knee more than that in the operating room before all the swelling had set in, and while you were asleep and could not feel it. The joint is fine, but there is plenty of swelling that keeps the knee from bending.

The physical therapist taught me to lift the foot of my operated leg off the floor by lifting my hip and swinging the leg forward as far as it would go until the heel rested on the floor. I don't think anyone who has a replacement knee forgets this lesson more than once. Once the operated leg was out of the way in front of me I could sit using just the good leg and my arms to lower myself onto the chair seat. Most often I landed on the front part of the seat and had to scoot back. Sitting on a straight chair without a footstool is just too painful at this point and I don't recommend it.

This summary of the general routine, by a man who had his replacement at Methodist Hospital in Omaha, sums up the experience most of us had.

The fifth floor staff at Methodist was exceptional. I had great care 24/7. The nurses were wonderful; the staff was caring and helpful. I had a program of rehab in the hospital. They had me up the day following surgery. Of course, I had had a spinal and femoral shot so pain was not an issue at that point. I was walked around the floor every day from Tuesday thru Thursday. I was 'tested' by a certified rehab person to be sure I could negotiate stairs, bathrooms, etc. before being released."

Living With A Knee Replacement

***

Physical Therapy: The Start of Recovery

Some people, including doctors, talk of physical therapy as torture. This is an unfair characterization. Physical therapy is painful, since moving the joint hurts, but it is hardly torture. These first sessions with the physical therapist allowed me, and will allow you, to take the first important steps in moving your new knee. Without the direction and support of the hospital physical therapy staff, I don't think I would have moved the knee as much as they showed me I could, even the day after surgery. In that first session in the gym, I did wonder if the therapist subscribed to the "physical therapy is torture" philosophy. I do note that he was the one and only person I came across in all my physical therapy who seemed to have that attitude.

Left to my own devices, I would have stayed in bed until released from the hospital, and maybe would have done the same thing at home. The knee would have stopped hurting, perhaps, but it would have gotten stiff and not had the flexibility it needed to get back to useful functioning.

My first physical therapy session on Tuesday morning had consisted of getting out of bed for the first time and taking a short walk to the door and back with the physical therapist walking alongside. The next session was in the afternoon and took place in the physical therapy gym. When the physical therapist came in the afternoon, he came with a wheelchair. I did enjoy it when the transportation person wheeled me down the halls. I had seen nothing but my room since I woke up. At Good

Samaritan Hospital the physical therapists came twice a day with the wheelchair. These visits were the real start of rehabilitation.

The gym was a large room. The center was open. There were platforms the size of a queen size bed, each topped with a thick foam mat lining the walls to the left and right. Patients, each attended by a physical therapist supervising their exercises and protecting them from harm, occupied some of the mats. Behind me was a parking lot for wheelchairs. The driver parked me in the lot and told me to wait.

The wait was not long. Soon a physical therapist appeared in front of me, stood my walker in front of me and told me to stand up. I braced myself on the arms of the wheelchair, pushed myself up with my good leg, and grasped the handles on the walker.

He pointed to the other end of the room where a set of parallel bars and a flight of three steps stood waiting. He told me to walk across the floor to the steps. And he didn't hold on to me. That was my first inkling that recovery was going to take a lot of work – on my part. For knee recipients the wheelchairs are only to get to and from the gym. Wheelchairs are not used inside the physical therapy gym.

The open room was pretty intimidating. I hobbled across the open space with my walker and stopped in front of the steps. I may have looked at the therapist with an expression that said, "I can't do that." Or I might have said it out loud. Maybe I just gulped. I can't remember.

At this juncture the only way to get up steps is to "one step" it, using the good leg to lift the body up to the next step and dragging the operated leg behind. Coming down is the opposite, leading with the operated leg and then lowering the body down with the good leg. These two simple tasks, walking across the room and going up a few steps, as difficult as they may seem at the time, give the patient confidence that he or she can recover from the surgery.

I remember being quite proud of myself when I got up and then down the steps without falling down.

The therapist guided me to one of the mats to work on exercises to start the process of straightening and bending the knee. The exercises have names like, "Ankle Pump" – bending the ankle up and down, and "Quad Set" -- tightening the thigh muscle with the leg lying straight on the bed. These two are easy even right after surgery.

Other exercises, those that are harder, have names like "Straight Leg Raise" – lifting the leg a few inches straight off the mat; "Short Arc Quad" – putting a rolled towel under the knee to bend it a little then trying to straighten the leg; "Long Arc Quad" – Sitting on the side of the bed with the knee bent at a ninety degree angle and then straightening the knee; and "Heel Slides" – Putting a strap under the heel while sitting on the mat and pulling the heel along the mat up toward the buttocks.

If you had exercises to do before the surgery to strengthen your leg these will be familiar.

Don't be concerned if you cannot do the more difficult exercises the first day. I couldn't do any of them. I almost screamed the first time the therapist put the towel under my knee for the short arc quads and let my knee bend enough for my heel to rest on the mat. I could not raise my leg an inch. With the first try at heel slides I may have gotten my knee bent twenty degrees, and that is not much. The long arc quads were the worse. I sat on the edge of the mat while the therapist held my leg straight out with his hand under my heel. The therapist began lowering my heel and I was almost instantly begging him to stop. He stopped well before he had bent my knee to a ninety degree angle. I could not raise my leg from where he supported it, not even a little. I felt pretty discouraged at that moment.

That is the physical therapy routine for Good Samaritan. Though Physical therapy is a part of the hospital routine at every hospital I am aware of, not all the programs are the same. I did not have occupational therapy while I was in the program.

Roxann, who had her surgery in Wisconsin, described the program at her hospital this way.

"The joint camp I mentioned was started by the orthopedic surgeons about six years ago to ease the transition from hospital surgery to home or wherever you had to go to rehab. All patients with joint replacements do go to joint camp. It also makes it easier for the surgeon to check on your progress daily if you are still in the hospital. Occupational Therapy did indeed come in and directed me in the set up of a daily hygiene program and dressing with some short cuts for ease of completion and safety. Physical Therapy came in and directed the use of the walker and walking in the walker safely. If you had steps to get into your home, they began to work with you on climbing a set of stairs. You only had to climb up and down a couple times the number of stairs you have in the home. I looked like a drunk hanging onto the rail and hoisting the old bod up those few stairs and looked the same once at home. Amazing how quickly strength came back even if not full!"

* * *

After that first session, I still had a lingering fear that something in the joint would come apart if anything jostled the joint. One incident dispelled that fear. The therapy aide had just wheeled me back to my room after a physical therapy session. The wheelchair had a footrest which elevated the operated leg so it did not bend to an angle which was painful. I was getting ready to transfer from the chair to my bed. I was looking forward to a good nap after a hard hour at therapy. The aide, a sweet young lady, reached down to support the operated leg and at the same time reached over to release the lever supporting the leg rest.

The footrest released before the aide had my leg in hand. I swear my leg quivered in mid-air. My wife said my heel bounced off the floor. I don't remember if I screamed or just ground my teeth. It did hurt a lot when the young lady dropped my leg; however, the extra pain was transient and did not last more than a few minutes. I was reassured with that proof that something so simple as being bounced off the floor would not damage the joint. In the end, the mortified aide needed more consoling than I did.

By late afternoon of this first day post surgery, all the chores; walking, washing up, sitting up, going to Physical therapy are over. There is time to lie in bed and try to read the newspaper or a book, visit with friends, watch TV or some other free time activity. Between the pain and the medication, you may find it hard to concentrate on anything you try to do. One person who has taken a lot of medication for pain said that morphine based pain killers, which is what you are probably taking, make all the muscles, including the eye muscles, relax and that makes focusing difficult. If you get a headache from not being able to focus for long, don't worry, there is nothing wrong with you.

Tuesday is a long day, with getting out of bed and then having a physical therapy session. You will have been encouraged to walk at other times. You will have sat up in the recliner, possibly for several hours in a row. You will probably have had visitors who came by to wish you well. The anesthetic from the operation will have completely worn off. In short, you will be tired.

Unfortunately, sleep may be slow or not come at all. After all you are in a strange environment and it's just not your bed. Sleep may be slow or not come. The knee, even with the painkillers will hurt some – or a lot. You've been on your back for most of several days and, if you are like me, cannot roll over onto your side or stomach. If you can roll over comfortably onto your side, or even do it without a great deal of pain, you are ahead of most patients. If you have the same experience as most knee replacement patients, you will spend an uncomfortable night trying to wiggle your buns into a comfortable position.

I found it actually helped to get up and go for a walk at 2:00 am. By my second surgery, I felt much more confident getting up on my own and strolling around with the walker. The hospital hallways are as quiet as Wal-Mart aisles at that time of night. Any staff you see smile as if they see someone gimping by in the middle of the night all the time. Actually, they do.

You might also try moving to the recliner, if you have one available, and watching TV rather than lying in bed tossing and turning through the night. I'm sure a nurse would be happy to put a blanket over you if you get cold.

THREE

WEDNESDAY: Life Restarts – Sort Of

The operated knee still has a lot of pain in it when someone, either you, the doctor, the nurse, or the physical therapist moves it. I spent a lot of time concentrating on not moving in any way that jostled the knee. The little pressure booties are still a nuisance. It's still awkward to eat a meal off the hospital tray. The IV cord gets in the way when you move your arm. And your backside is still exposed by the open air hospital gowns you have had to wear. You may be lucky and have one of the more humane wrap around gowns that tie in the front. Other than that, it is just like any other day in the hospital.

Many of the knee recipients I talked to felt strong enough to get in and out of bed independently on Wednesday. If you find you are not able to manage it on your own, ask for as much help as you need. The joint is stable but a fall would not do any good.

One recipient told me she knew a woman in her late sixties who fell on her new knee and shattered her femur. I don't know how true her story is, but I did not want to have a fall and find out what would happen. I mentioned that story to my therapist who said such an injury would be very uncommon. He suspected, if the story were true, that there was an underlying cause such as poor bone density.

Most recipients have become well aware that the pain from the surgery is not getting less. Almost everyone is familiar with the pain that comes from a cut or a bruise. With a cut or bruise the pain starts to ease up in a few days and disappears over a week or so. With replacement surgery, the sharp pain which we usually associate with "I've been hurt", lasts much longer. Remember, the surgeon had to cut away several slabs of bone to fit the new joint, and bone pain lasts longer than pain in the soft tissues. Those who have had a knee replacement have all experienced the long lasting fiery pain that comes whenever they move.

The pain can build up even when you are lying perfectly still. I remember many times in the first weeks when I was lying perfectly still and the knee began to throb and ache more and more and more. Sometimes shifting to a new position helped. Other times I had to just bear with it.

Remember, the grinding, exhausting pain of bone on bone you had for years does not exist any more. That source of pain is gone. The prosthetic joint separates the bone ends from each other, and all the friction of standing or walking is borne by your bright shiny new knee. Okay, maybe the parts are no longer as bright and shiny as they were the day the surgeon installed them. It's still a great image for the new joint. In spite of the fiery pain in the first few weeks the recipient can confidently walk on the joint and safely bend it as far as the pain and swelling allow.

With all the talk of pain it's a wonder anyone actually goes through with the surgery. Perhaps part of the reason any recipient agrees to the operation is that he or she does not know how much it would hurt. Even so, six months after the first surgery, I had the other knee done. Only six months after I had the first knee replaced, the minor pains were much less than the agony I had before surgery. The pain from the operation is different from the grinding, exhausting pain that I endured for years with the worn out knee joints. The pain from the surgery is "clean" and sharp. There is something that seems healthy in how the knee hurts after surgery.

Sometime in the morning, before the shower, a nurse came in and removed the IV from the back of my hand. From then on I had to ask for pain medication when it got too bad.

You may experience the treat of taking a shower on this second day post surgery. For most of us, in our normal, real life, a shower signals that the day has started, and it certainly makes one feel better to wash off two days of gunk. After two days without bathing a shower just feels "normal."

One of the hardest things about showering for me was accepting that the water would not hurt the incision. The staples hold the skin together quite well, and the skin is already starting to mend.

One woman talked about the difficulty stepping over the three inch tall lip of the shower stall. That did not stop her. She said several student nurses were helping her at the time. She said she hurt so bad she did not care if her behind was showing but still kept apologizing to the student nurses.

Some hospitals will have nice big showers with handrails and plenty of room for a stool to sit on. Unfortunately the joint wing at the hospital where I had my surgeries is in an older part of the hospital, and the shower stalls were barely large enough for me much less a stool. When I looked in the shower stall and saw most of the room taken up by a small stool, I chose to evict the stool and painfully stand on my good leg for the few minutes it took to wash off, while I prayed I didn't fall over. Though I could only stand for a few minutes it felt good to be clean. And it was a great morale booster to do something normal.

I spoke to one gentleman who had his surgery in the same hospital as I did. He did manage to sit on the little stool in the tiny shower stall, though he said it hurt like heck. That he was able to sit is proof that the knee actually will bend somewhat more than I was willing to tolerate. In other words, he was a lot tougher than I was.

You may feel pretty wobbly and it is smart to take as much help as is needed in getting into and out of the shower.

After a shower it is time to dress. You have probably only worn the open back hospital gown you wore into surgery, or one like it. I don't remember if I had a clean gown between the surgery and the shower, but my memory was a bit fuzzy. Dressing in something other than a hospital gown is another one of those normal things that boosts morale. Unfortunately, dressing is not easy. I had to sit down on the water-closet to dress. The hospital bed was too high and not at all private.

The easiest clothes to put on at this stage are loose and comfy. My wife bought a nice jogging suit with zippers at the bottom of the legs so I didn't have to try to squeeze my swollen knee into the jeans I wore when I came to the hospital. The only place you will be going in the next few days is home so there is no one to impress.

Dressing starts with the operated leg. If you are a double replacement it's a toss up whether to start with the left or right side. I'd bet that you start with the same side you usually did before the surgery. People are creatures of habit. The first thing I noticed when I tried to get my drawers on was that I could not lift the foot of my operated leg off the floor. I had to lean way forward with my arms stretched out and sort of drop my drawers over my toes and hang on to them with one hand. Since I couldn't lift my heel it was a matter of dragging the waistline under the heel of the operated leg. I could lift the foot of the good leg just enough to slip the waist under the heel, though if I tried to lift the leg very far it felt like I was going to topple over. Mostly, I sort of draped my underwear and pants over my feet and prayed.

Once the underwear and pants were over my feet and pulled up past my knees, I could stand up and pull everything the rest of the way up. It's easier to do both at one time rather than going through the process of sitting and standing twice.

The easy part of dressing is putting on a shirt. Since both arms work fine, it is easy to do. The only caution is that you have to watch your balance a bit.

Pulling socks on was more than I could manage. The whole time I was in the hospital I let the nurse manage the standard issue non-slip socks. It was not a burden for the nurse since she had to come in and let me out of the pressure booties every time I wanted to get out of bed.

Physical therapy continued with morning and afternoon sessions. The routine was the same each time; walk across the floor, climb the stairs, then do the same exercises I had done the first day. Each time you do the exercises it will hurt but the muscles gain strength and movement each day. By the second day of physical therapy I could move my operated leg a little even during the accursed long arc quad exercise. That's the one sitting on the edge of the mat when, the first day, I begged the therapist to stop. Really, I begged him to stop during each session, but each time he lowered my foot a little more.

At this early point in recovery, the knee recipient needs to make a commitment to work hard to do the exercises in physical therapy and get the joint moving. From what I could gather the doctor will not release the patient until he or she thinks it will be safe for the patient to go home. The physical therapy people are snitches by the way, so working hard for them is in your best interests.

On Wednesday, the Good Samaritan Joint Replacement program held a special lunch for that week's joint replacement patients. We had four knees and two hips the week I was in. The purpose of the meeting was to brief the patients on what they would need to do, from a medical perspective, when they went home. The main topics were pain medications, stool softeners (because of the pain

50

medications), how to administer the blood thinners (to prevent clots), and other medical stuff.

The lunch was well intentioned provided good advice about medication issues when we left the comfortable confines of the hospital. Also, it felt good to be a part of the group. The Wednesday luncheon was the only time the joint replacement patients got together, though we were all in the same wing of the hospital. One recipient remembered seeing fliers for the luncheon in her room, "but did not read them as I was so doped up." Another said someone wheeled her in without telling her what was going on, or she was so groggy she forgot they had told her. Another said she came in directly from physical therapy and was already tired.

The problem I had was that the meeting was in a conference room with the usual straight back conference room chairs. My knee still did not bend well enough to sit comfortably in a straight chair. Several of the knee patients found the pain of sitting so great that, after about thirty minutes they became nauseous and thought they were going to pass out. I was one of those who couldn't take it and left early. If your hospital has this kind of a program in a regular conference room ask for a footstool to elevate your leg.

The program information is good, but it was hard to remember what was being said when I was hurting so much, and was still pretty groggy with the pain meds. I suggest bringing someone with you to take notes. The information is important for medical care when at home. Fortunately, my wife was able to get away from her work and come with me. It's a good thing she read all the hospital literature, or I would have forgotten everything.

Other than physical therapy sessions, or a special program like the luncheons, the knee recipient is on his or her own to sleep - something most of us did a lot, watch TV, read - if they can concentrate, or entertain visitors. You will be encouraged to be up in a chair more each day. Sitting up helps prevent pneumonia by letting the lungs work easier. And sitting helps keep your muscles in shape after days in bed.

You will be encouraged to be up and walking around the halls two or three times a day on your own. Even though walking was painful and I didn't feel very steady with the walker at times, I enjoyed the feeling of being upright. With each walk I took, I could feel some strength coming back. I was encouraged that I could do it on my own, no matter how halting it seemed to me at the time. If walking is difficult or you feel unsteady you can get someone to walk beside you for safety.

In the afternoon my oxygen levels had stabilized enough that the oxygen cannula was no longer necessary. I was glad not to have a tube up my nose. I did notice that I had a sore throat for a time after the cannula was gone. It nurse said that was normal.

By the end of the day most recipients are free from the intravenous needle and the oxygen hookup. With the IV gone the patient has to ask for a pill when the pain gets bad. Not everyone was happy to have the magic button gone. Ed, who was sixty-one the year he had both knees done, had this to say. "They take you off the drip after two days and start the pill. How often do you take those things, every two hours – four hours? After three hours you're about ready to bend the rails on the bed." He clenched his fist is mid air to demonstrate.

Most recipients will be eating if they have been having trouble with nausea from the anesthesia. If you are fortunate and your doctor thinks you are moving around enough, he or she will order the pressure booties discontinued when you are in bed – Aaah! It was so nice to be in bed and not have my feet strapped to the foot of the bed. I still did not sleep well at night, but my feet were free.

FOUR

THURSDAY: They Let You Go Home – HOORAY!

If everything has gone according to plan, this is going home day for most knee recipients. I woke up with all the tubes and needles removed. I knew that I was going home today and looked forward to eating breakfast. Some patients may have a longer stay due to a medical condition or some problem that arises. Usually, a longer stay is not a surprise as the knee recipient and their doctor will have agreed that a longer stay is necessary - necessary, perhaps, but not desired. I did not talk to one knee replacement patient who said they begged to stay in the hospital longer. I think most of us figured if we were going to suffer we might as well suffer in our own beds.

Getting ready to go home is wonderful. By the third day, maybe with just a little help, you can get out of bed, take a quick shower and get dressed. I say "quick", but that may only refer to how long you stay in the shower.

Everything you do will seem to be in slow motion. Shoes and socks will still be a pesky problem.

If you are brave you might try to push your toes into a pair of loose slip-ons. It hurts a bit when you push with the operated leg, but it does feel like an accomplishment the first time you can wiggle your toes into shoes. I managed the feat with some old deck shoes then vowed not to put shoes on again for a few days. As soon as I was home I put away everything but my slippers. The next time I tried shoes was two weeks later.

Before you leave the hospital, a nurse will instruct you how to give yourself an injection of blood thinner medication. This medicine is important to prevent blood clots forming around the knee and working their way to the lungs or heart. The idea of giving yourself a shot might be pretty spooky. The needle is really fine, meaning thin, it doesn't hurt, and it is short. The technique is not complicated. You pinch the skin on your stomach by your belly-button, poke the needle straight in and push the plunger. If you take the opportunity to practice giving yourself a shot in the hospital with a nurse to guide you, you will get a great confidence booster for when you have to do it at home.

Packing up is a happy time. I suggest watching while whoever is taking you home gathers your belongings. They may have quite an armload. There are all the things you brought with you when you came to the hospital. Then there all the items you acquired while you were a patient; the plastic breathing device, box of tissues, urinal (which you might need for a few days), ice pack (which you will definitely use for a month or more), gait belt (helpful for heel slide exercise), and everything else. My wife had so much to carry that I wound up holding my walker while a hospital aide pushed me to the front door in a wheelchair.

All hospitals, as far as I can tell, insist on wheeling the patient out the front door. Maybe the administration does not want anyone falling down and breaking something after they have just vacated a bed.

My wife brought the car around while I waited eagerly with the aide who wheeled me down to the front door. When the car was in place at the pick up area in front of the hospital, the aide showed me another trick, how to get into the car. The trick worked well, though I looked something like a wounded duck doing it. I spoke to several knee recipients whose nurse simply left them at the curb with no instructions.

Here's how the trick works. One helper slides the passenger seat as far back as possible. Then they lay the seatback down as far as it will go. You stand up from the wheelchair next to the open car door, swivel around until your rear end is toward the seat, kick the operated leg forward, and lower your self down on the edge of the seat. The next step is to use your arms to lift and scrunch your butt in as far as possible. I was almost sitting on the center console. Now comes the fun part. Using trick one or having someone lift the operated leg swing the leg into the car bending the knee just enough to squeeze the toes in. Now you can ease down into the seat, while your helper raises the seatback so you can look out the window instead of just staring at the roof.

The last step is to give a big sigh of relief. You are no longer a patient, just someone going home to recover.

Right then it was easy for me to smile and wave goodbye to hospital and the aide who had brought me down to freedom.

FIVE

HOME AGAIN

Here is a warning. You will be amazed at how many bumps there are in the road between the hospital and your front door. Every one of these bumps hurts, or at least sends twinges of pain up the operated leg. The bumps and consequent pain jolts make it a little hard to appreciate the ride home. The bumping around does no harm to the leg, it just hurts when the injured bones and swollen tissues bounce around.

Ask your driver not to make any sudden stops. Two weeks after my first operation we went to a granddaughter's baptism in a town an hour away. On the way home, my wife had to slam on the brakes to avoid someone who ran a red light. I'm pretty sure I screamed that time.

Getting out of the car is the reverse of getting in and is just as awkward. The car door or grab bars are great supports to hoist yourself to your feet from the car seat. Make sure your driver has the walker in place by the open car door before you start to stand up.

Actually getting into the house may seem daunting. There are very few homes which have no steps on the way in. I was glad I had the practice going up and down steps during physical therapy at the hospital. The three steps going into my house did not have a railing. I was able to set the walker ahead of me on the landing then hold onto the doorframe to negotiate the first two steps. The same technique worked for the final step into the kitchen. I really appreciated my wife's willingness to risk her own safety by standing behind me in case I lost my balance and fell back. We had no contingency plan for if I fell forward.

My doctor cautioned me not to go up too many stairs at first, and not to attempt full flights of stairs for a while. The advice was good. I was too weak to try managing a whole flight of stairs. And my balance was pretty shaky. Fortunately, I live in a ranch home, and did not have to go into the basement living area until I was ready.

If the main living area in your house is on two floors you might want to schedule your day so you don't have to manage the stairs for more than one round trip a day. One recipient, who lives in a tri-level home, set up a sleeping area on the main floor for several weeks until she had recovered enough to manage stairs better.

At first going up steps is hard. It is a challenge to lift the leg. All of us started doing stairs by stepping up with the good leg and lifting the operated leg onto the same step, then repeating the process, the same "one stepping" you did in the physical therapy gym at the hospital. Going down stairs is definitely a one step at a time deal. Step down with your operated leg, bending the knee of your good leg to lower yourself. The quadriceps muscle on the operated leg is not yet strong enough to control the descent. My physical therapist said that the quadriceps muscle is responsible for both stepping up and stepping down but it works differently for each task.

Once I was in the house my thought process was, "Home, bed!" Getting dressed, riding home, and getting into the house were tiring. Resting is highly recommended. I headed for my bed. If your home base is your bed I suggest pulling the covers free at the foot of the bed and turning them back toward the center. With the covers out of the way it is much easier to lift the operated leg up and in the bed. It is a simple matter to throw the covers back over the leg.

Not everyone will be comfortable in their bed at this point. Some knee recipients make their home base a sofa or a recliner. One lady slept on a couch for the first two weeks after she found her bed a little too high to lift her leg onto it.

Most of us, now that we were home, wanted to get rid of everything that was a nuisance. The ice pack certainly seems to qualify. It is bulky, cold and has to be changed every four or five hours. Do not stop using the ice. The tissues around your new knee are terribly swollen and the ice pack is simply your best ally to help reduce the swelling.

When you climb in bed put the ice pack on your knee, and leave it there – all day and all night. Take it with you when you move from your bed to your chair and back again. A good rule is that you have to the ice pack on your knee except when you are on the pot, walking or doing exercises. If the ice feels too cold, you might put a towel between your skin and the ice pack. I used a towel frequently at night so I could get some sleep. The hospital sent me home with a fabric sleeve that held chemical ice packs. There was an extra set of the chemical packs so there was always a cold set available.

For the first few days my wife was in charge of changing out the ice packs when they lost their cool. A few days later, when I could drape the fabric sleeve of the ice packs over the front bar of the walker and carry it to the kitchen to change out the thawed chemical packs with the ones from the freezer she told me that I wasn't a cripple and could do it myself. I loved that Paula encouraged me to do those things I could.

One last thing before going to bed is the blood thinners. I usually gave myself the shot while in bed. It just seemed easier to get hold of a pinch of skin on my stomach while lying down because I didn't have to concentrate on giving myself the shot and standing up at the same time.

The last activity of that first day was turning in for the night. I wish I could tell you that being home and in your own bed will make you sleep like a baby. Unfortunately, no one I talked to had that experience. We all found it difficult to sleep through the night. Many reported more pain at night, probably because of the human tendency to focus more on our pain when other activities during the day distract us. Lying in one spot for hours also seems to cause the operated knee to throb/ache/hurt, etc.

Living With A Knee Replacement

The knee recipients I talked to report an array of strategies for trying to get some sleep. One lady slept on a couch in the living room. She lay on her side with her own back to the back of the couch and a pillow between her legs. She hugged another pillow to keep from rolling off the couch.

Portrait of a recovering knee recipient.

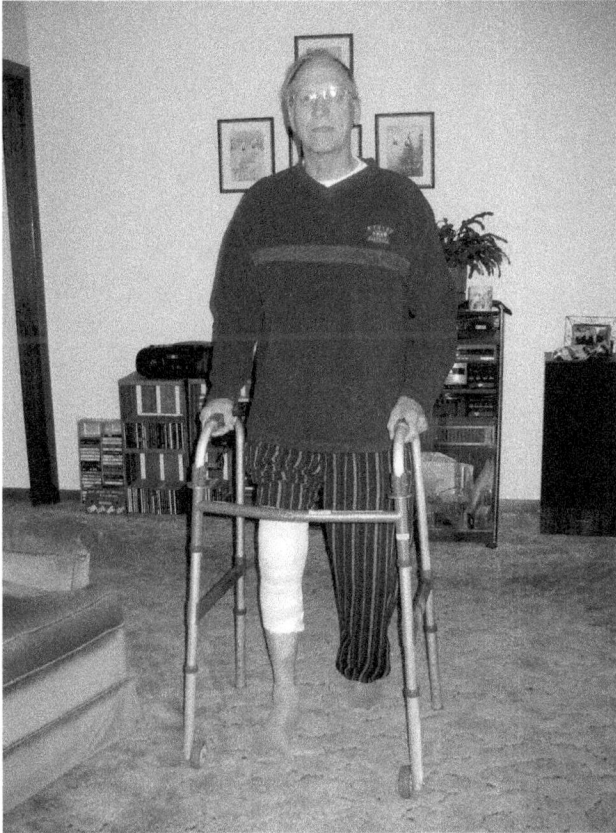

I hobbled around the house like this for a week. The bandage shows clearly. The light area below is where all the hair was shaved. Normally, I had my pants leg pulled down. Notice my expression is not too grim. You can see I did have a lot of bad hair days. Recting and taking care of yourself will take precedence over neatness at this point in recovery.

PART TWO

BEND IT

(Weeks two through four or six)

I think all of us who have had a knee replacement would have been happy if we could have gone home from the hospital and been able to say, "Well, that's over now I can go on with my life." It does not work that way.

When a knee replacement owner goes home it is only the start of a long journey of recovery from a serious operation that has left him or her weak and hurting. The good news is that the owner does not have to stay in the hospital the whole time of recovery, or even the week that was common in the past. After a few days the owner will be able to hobble around the house on their own.

The main emphasis of recovery at this stage is to manage the pain and to start bending the knee. If the owner does not bend the knee it may not work for them as well as they would like when fully recovered.

During this time the owner will be able to settle into a routine around the house and get started caring for his or her self while returning to normal.

SIX

SETTLING IN AT HOME

If the last few paragraphs sound like a prescription to go home and lie in bed, they are not. Your doctor allowing you to go home from the hospital is the signal the operation was successful. Now it is time to focus on the first main task of recovery, bending the knee so you get used to using it.

Waking up the second day at home is much like waking up in the hospital. The operated leg still does not bend. The knee is still stiff and achy. The pain will probably have kept you up most of the night, no matter where or how you tried to sleep. The good news is that you will wake up in your own house with your own things around you, and no one poking you for blood samples at five o'clock in the morning. All these things are small comforts.

The morning will start slow. Stiffness comes during the night and balance is shakiest first thing in the morning. It might be a good idea to keep the urinal handy for a day or two. However, you do need to get up and start moving. The sooner you start moving the knee in the morning, the sooner it loosens up. My routine at first was to get up for the bathroom and then climb back in bed, where my wife served breakfast on a tray until I started my exercises.

Most of us went home on our own, trusting ourselves to whoever we had agreed to take care of us. For me it was my wife, Paula. Another knee replacement patient, Mike, had a different scenario. "The Visiting Nurses Association was contracted to my care. Each day they came to inspect the knee, bandage, temp, swelling, etc. as well as blood tests to be sure the blood thinner was correct."

I did not talk to anyone who had any problems with those issues. Though, if you are on your own, and have any concerns at all, please get in touch with your doctor to see if there is a problem.

* * *

Exercises – The Work Starts

When I had my very first knee surgery to rebuild the right knee twenty-five years ago, the patient next to me was a knee replacement patient. He shared his bed with a contraption which slowly bent and straightened his knee – all day and all night. From what I can gather it was a painful process that went on for a week in the hospital. The machine insured the patient's knee kept moving so it did not lock up. Today's instructions to walk and do exercises serve the same purpose, though now the patient has to hold his or her self accountable and not let a machine do all the work.

My therapist told stories of knee recipients who did not keep the knee moving and had to go back into surgery so the doctor could bend the knee and break up the adhesions – scar tissue. He said no one could stand the pain without anesthesia. I sure did not want to find out.

My knee replacement team sent me home with the instruction to walk at least two-hundred feet three times a day. For me, that was three laps from the bedroom to the kitchen. The first few days it was a tough chore. Three times a day, I had to move my leg off the bed – ouch. Then I had to round up the walker and stand on my leg – ouch. Then I had to step and step and step all the way to the kitchen - ouch. Before the operation the trip had seemed short. Now, it seemed like walking across country. With the kitchen as a destination, I had an excuse to pick up a cookie. There are not many things more motivating for me than cookies.

Every doctor seems to have a little different routine. One lady, along with the exercises, had the prescription to take a ten minute walk three times a day instead of having a distance specified.

My prescription was to do ten repetitions of the exercises that I had done in physical therapy at the hospital three times a day. I thought it was easier to take a walk first to loosen up, and then do the exercises.

When I was done with one of the walks and exercises I could sink back in bed and take a nap. I scheduled the walk and exercise sessions for morning, afternoon and evening. My wife complimented me frequently on how faithful I was in doing the exercises. More than once her encouragement was the only thing that got me out of bed.

One lady, who was on Medicare, had an order from her doctor for a Home-Health nurse to come in daily to help with the exercises.

The sets of exercises are painful and difficult at first. The first few weeks you may be saying to yourself, "No way, it hurts too much." But doing the exercises prescribed from the hospital, consistently and purposefully is the only sure way to get back on your feet. The props for the exercises are easy to come by; a rolled up towel, a coffee can wrapped in a towel, and the gait belt the hospital sent home (a towel or belt will also work.)

The hardest of the exercises the long arc quad, sitting on the edge of the bed and trying to straighten the knee, this is the same exercise that gave me trouble in the hospital. I have vivid memories of sitting on the edge of my bed feeling the pain above my knee from trying to contract the muscle and watching my leg not move. I wondered what would happen if my leg never moved. It did move, a little at first, and then more each time I tried. It was a week before I could straighten my leg even once. The second hardest exercise was the heel slide, sitting on the bed and pulling the foot toward the buttocks with a towel or belt. At least with the heel slide there was movement. Even though these exercises are hard, working on them now pays off in the end.

Living With A Knee Replacement

* * *

The two weeks following surgery will settle into a routine of trying to get comfortable napping, doing exercises, taking meds and eating. Television may play a big part in the day, and maybe some light reading. It's hard to concentrate in the first few weeks, so don't plan on doing heavy brain work. The body needs a lot of rest and doing the most routine things, eating, showering, dressing, and such are more tiring than most of us expected.

For the first few days my dear wife brought my meals to me, so I did not have to get up again. I enjoyed getting my meals in bed or in my recliner. There is a practical reason for taking meals in bed or a recliner for the first few days. It is just impossible to sit comfortably in a kitchen chair. First, you have to sit on the front edge of the chair because your knee does not bend enough to let you push back. So, your back starts to hurt. Then the backs of your thighs press on the edge of the chair which makes them hurt. Last, the operated leg hangs down at a semi-bent angle and makes the knee throb. Trying to sit is an altogether unpleasant experience.

Most of the knee recipients I talked to still found it hard to concentrate long enough to read or watch TV. Remember you are still taking those painkillers which relax all of your muscles. The narcotic pain pills might also account for some of the frequent naps. A common occurrence with me was to start out reading or watching TV and wake up several hours later. Then I might be awake for another hour or two and disappear into another nap. The body just needs rest to heal and sleeping is an important part of getting that rest.

The swelling does not seem to go down much in this time. The pain continues at a high level, and the knee still hurts like fire. That initial fiery pain lasts for two or three weeks. There is nothing to do about it. The bones which have been insulted in the surgery need to heal. The good news is there is no pain in the actual knee joint since there are no longer any nerves there. In spite of the pain, the best thing to do is continue walking on the new knee and doing your exercises just as the doctor ordered. Most of the knee recipients I spoke to had the same experience and time lines.

I am not the only one who had flashbacks of, "What did I let them do to me?" Hang on. It does get better.

Here is a warning. It is hard to carry things when using a walker or crutches. Some things, like pillows, blankets and ice bags, you can drape over the front bar of the walker. Coffee cups and plates are a "no go" until you are walking on your own. I did figure out I could carry a bowl, then the cereal box, and finally the milk jug to the table and assemble my cereal after I sat down. I never did figure out how to carry a cup of coffee or a glass of milk when I was using the walker.

Standing and walking balance is shaky simply because the quadriceps muscle shut down as a result of the surgery. I had more trouble with balance when the room was dark. People use visual cues to help with balance. When these cues are absent, the body has to rely on its internal balance mechanism, which surgery temporarily upsets. The upset leads to problems with balance. Be sure of your balance before trying to walk. Fortunately, I did not fall, but am sure I would not have been able to get up if I had.

Blankets, pillows, clothes, shoes, newspapers, and anything else lying on the floor represent hazards. You simply are not able to lift the foot of the operated leg over such obstacles. One double knee recipient told of how nice it was the day she was able to step over a hose stretched across her driveway. For her that red letter day came about two months after surgery. You might want to leave a nightlight on till you feel more secure.

In the first few weeks of recovery there are only a few places you are likely to want to go; to the bathroom, from one resting place to another, on the thrice daily walks around the house, and possibly to the kitchen to try to sit in a chair long enough to eat a meal.

The first obstacle you face on the way to the bathroom may be the width of the door. Standard bathroom doors are not as wide as a walker. To get into the bathroom with my walker I had to turn the walker sideways then scuttle sideways through the door like a crab. Also, allow plenty of time. You are moving more slowly than you usually do. I find as I get older my bladder does not give me as much warning as it used to.

The second obstacle is the toilet seat. It is only about fifteen inches high, where chairs are nineteen inches high. Those four inches make a big difference when your knee does not bend very well.

It helps to have a sturdy counter nearby to use as a lever to get down to the seat and up again. Do not use your towel bar. A towel bar usually mounts only in the drywall and will pull off the wall if you put a lot of weight on it. If getting up and down is too much, you can get a riser to temporarily mount on the toilet seat. You can talk to the case manager at the hospital to arrange for a riser before you leave the hospital if you think you will need one. You might also rent one from a medical supply store or even purchase one.

A lady recipient said she used a riser with handles on the side. She recommends it for all female knee replacement recipients. She is saving the one she bought for when she has her second knee done in another few months.

Lowering your pants only down to your knee makes it easier to kick the operated leg out using trick two. As for getting comfortable on the seat with one leg sticking out and your pants at your knees, that is something each knee recipient has to figure out in the privacy of his or her own bathroom. I could not find a way to sit comfortably, until I was well along in healing. I usually wound up sitting canted away from the operated leg.

There is another issue on using the commode. Most recipients will be taking narcotic pain medication. The medicine causes constipation. Even with the stool softeners, prescribed to counteract the effects of the narcotic pain medication, having a bowel movement may be hard until you are finished with the narcotic pain meds.

Sleeping is another issue that you will have to deal with. Most nights I started trying to sleep in my bed. I am one who has always slept on his side, so I may have had more trouble than people who usually sleep on their back. When I was not able to fall asleep in bed, I moved to my recliner and watched old movies till the wee hours when I usually dozed off for a few hours.

After the first surgery a friend moved a recliner next to my bed. I think having me moving around from bed to recliner when I could not sleep nearly drove Paula crazy. After a week I had the friend move the recliner to the next room.

Looking back I had started taking more naps during the day long before I thought of actually having my knees replaced. The naps were to compensate for the exhaustion caused by the pain of my bad knees.

When the recliner did not work, I would move to the couch in the living room. On rare nights the pain was so great that all I could do was lie on the couch and moan through the night. My wife thought some of the reason I could not sleep at night was that I was sleeping too much during the day. I respect her opinions but on this I think she was wrong.

After a couple weeks I was able to fall asleep in bed but woke after a few hours. Then it was back to the recliner and more old movies. After three or four weeks I was awake more during the day and able to sleep more at night.

My wife changed the dressings on my knee every day. Changing the dressing is something you will need help with. Whoever is changing the dressing has to pull the sleeve which holds the gauze pads in place down to the ankle. It is just too hard for the patient to bend the knee far enough to reach that far. My wife helped with changing the dressing until I had the staples removed and no longer needed a dressing. She liked to see how the wound was healing, even though there did not seem to be much change for a while.

Taking a shower at home is another new experience. I could not step into the tub to take a shower. If you have a walk in shower, you are ahead of the game. Those of us who have a regular tub have a problem. One knee recipient told me she would stand in front of the tub trying to figure out how she was going to get her leg in.

For the first week I had a plastic stool in the tub. It cost a few dollars at the discount store. Paula supported me while I backed up to the tub and sat on the stool. It was scary to sit on the wobbly stool. This is a time to have all the help you might need. Then I did trick one to get my legs into the tub.

I was able to lean forward far enough to pull the shower knob up and divert the water from the tub to the shower head. I was careful to adjust the temperature before that step since I was in no position to jump out of the way if the water was scalding or freezing. The hospital showers had been a quick wash off as I was afraid of standing very long. It felt good to be able to sit and let the water run over me.

Getting out of the tub was the reverse process. Swing the legs out of the tub and then stand up from the stool. My wife was gracious enough to stay in the bathroom and help me by making sure the walker was in place and giving me support while I stood. After a few days I felt more secure and was able to do the whole operation myself. Remember the instruction you received when you took your first shower in the hospital, "Pat the incision dry and don't rub it."

After the shower I would finish my grooming while leaning against the counter as a concession to poor balance and tiredness. Then it was dress in "comfies" (what we, in our house, call the most comfortable clothes we can find) and back to bed for a nice rest. I never tried a tub bath but think it would have been nearly impossible to lower myself all the way into the tub. If I had been able to lower myself into the tub, I would never have been able to get out.

By the end of the first week at home, I had learned the trick of swinging the operated knee out to the side and over the tub edge, while leaning on the wall for support. Shower rods are just as likely as towel bars to pull off the wall, so they are not good for support. I also made sure there was a non slip mat in the bottom of the tub. For a few days I still sat on the stool in the tub until I got brave enough to stand through the shower. I felt pretty grown up when I could take a shower without supervision.

Also, during this time when I was spending so much time lying on my back I noticed a terrible itching developing. When Paula investigated, she found I had a nasty rash developing on my back. She was gracious enough to put lotion on the rash several times a day. The lotion helped the itching but the rash did not really go away until I was up more.

During the second week I was able to bend down and pull a sock over my toes then pull it up. I was also able to switch from slippers and loose slip-ons.

Not everything went on in the house. When Paula thought I could scuttle around the house pretty well, she suggested I go outside for a walk. After a few weeks in the house, I was eager for a change in scenery. When she got home from work in the evening she would go out with me for a walk on the street in front of the house. I had to manage the three steps in the front of the house. Like every new trick it was scary, but if you go slow and are careful getting out is worth the effort.

I would have liked to have seen me shuffling down the street, behind my walker, dressed in my sweat suit and slippers. I had given up the walker in the house but used it outside where the ground was not so even. The first time out I made it a half block before turning around. As the days passed the walks got a little longer, until I could make it a whole block. When I was done a nap was in order.

Every new trick was a treat. I do want to stress that you should get as much help as needed to keep from falling, though your recovery will be faster and better if you keep trying to do as much for yourself as you are able.

SEVEN

FREEDOM – THE STAPLES ARE GONE

About ten to fourteen days post surgery a new stage of healing begins. That is when you go for a visit to your surgeon's office or a home health nurse comes in, and the staples come out. Whether it hurts to have the staples removed depends on who you ask. The response, when given by the person who takes the staples out, ranges from "This won't hurt" to "This may sting a little." The nurse who removed my staples said it is better to have a nurse remove the staples because doctors aren't as be gentle as nurses. There might just be a little professional pride talking in that piece of advice. When the patient answers, the answer ranges from "Ouch!" to "Geez that hurts" to "Get away from me with that staple puller." I come down on the side of the patient.

The device used to remove surgical staples is not like the staple puller on your desk. The staple puller is a little device the size of a pair of tweezers with two arms sticking out in front. The arms slide under each end of the staple. When whoever is removing your stitches squeeze the handle, a third arm descends on the middle of the staple from above. The top arm is supposed to bend the staple in the middle so its two legs slide smoothly out of the skin. It doesn't always work that way. Sometimes the legs of the staples have gotten stuck in the skin, and drag the skin along with them when they come out. Even if the staple hurts when it comes out there will be only a drop of blood if any. Most of the staples come out pretty smoothly with no blood and no big ouch.

The most graphic description was from the lady who said that when the staples came out it felt like they were taking pieces of flesh with them. It just feels that way.

It seems miraculous that when all of the staples are out the skin the incision stays stuck together. The first sensation I had was one of relief. The staples are no longer there to pull on the skin each time that you move your knee. Once the staples are out there is no longer a need for a dressing on the incision. You will be able to walk out of the doctor's office knowing that the incision, your incision, will not open up again. It is satisfying to have all the extra hardware gone.

Scott, the Certified Athletic Trainer who oversaw my rehab in physical therapy told me that range of motion, how much the knee will bend, seems to improve in a hurry once the staples are out. The reason may be as simple as the fact that the staples are no longer pulling on the skin and causing discomfort. I would not argue with that theory.

The scar looks pretty ugly. After all, the wound from the incision is not yet two weeks old. A lot of scar tissue has built up around the site of the incision. Our human instinct is to let it alone so it can heal. Scott and another denizen of the physical therapy gym, a hockey player who had gone through several rehabs following knee surgeries, recommended using Vitamin E, applied as oil or as a lotion, to reduce the scar. I used the concentrated oil.

Just rub the oil or lotion on the scar and use your fingers to massage back and forth at a ninety degree angle across the line of the scar. Use as much pressure as you can tolerate and work your fingers up and down the scar once or twice. It feels pretty weird but does not hurt. One recipient said that a home health nurse told her to wait until all the scabs were gone before working on the scar.

The idea is that the vitamin E softens the tissue and the friction breaks up the scar tissue. I used the vitamin E for six or eight weeks until I could not tell that the scar was getting any smaller.

After the first application I noticed the excess oil stained the pajamas I was wearing. After that I wiped off the excess oil after I was finished massaging the scar and had no more problems.

In six months the scar was down to a pink line that was somewhat noticeable. In nine months there was only a thin white line that is barely noticeable. No one ever commented on the scar when I was wearing shorts n the summer, so it is no big deal. I am a little disappointed, though, since I like to brag a little about my new knees.

A quick search on the internet will turn up any number of creams and treatments for scars. Some of them might be useful and others probably fit under the heading of *snakeoil*. I just went with something I could get handily at the corner pharmacy.

EIGHT

PHYSICAL THERAPY – MAKING IT HURT

(Or, if it doesn't hurt you're not moving it.)

When my doctor referred me to physical therapy, he said with no trace of humor, "Well, I'm sending you over to be tortured." That line surely did not help my confidence any. I thought I was already hurting enough without being tortured. Why did I need to go for more pain? I remembered how much the brief physical therapy in the hospital hurt the first few times I had to use the muscles around the knee again. Why go? Because it speeds healing and physical therapy is not torture.

Most of the people I met who went to physical therapy went for four to six weeks depending on how fast they came along.

An unexpected benefit of going to physical therapy sessions came from the encouragement of the staff at the physical therapy clinic and the camaraderie of the other people recovering from injuries and surgery.

The most common question that comes up in therapy according to Scott, who was my trainer in physical therapy, is, "When is the pain going to stop?" Therapy may feel like torture when the patient's mind is on having the pain stop, and the therapeutic activities are focused on getting the joint functional – which causes pain. All I can say is that the pain of the surgery is different than the pain of moving the joint. On this point I have to just say, "Trust me."

Physical therapy is a topic of some disagreement among physicians. One lady's experience sums it up. Bennie, who was sixty when she had her knee replaced, writes, "I discovered that not all doctors prescribe physical therapy – my doctor didn't. I had to ask for it. My doctor's Physician's Assistant told me I didn't need it – I could do it on my own at home. He said they didn't always prescribe physical therapy for their patients. He said they have to weigh cost vs. benefit and they have seen some patients injured by having too aggressive physical therapy. He said they have to watch costs – insurance costs."

Mike did his rehab at home, though he had someone actively follow his progress.

"I rented a device to mechanically raise and lower my leg/knee which I used multiple times a day. My rehab therapist was in every other day to take me through exercises to build muscle strength, stretching and mobility.

"I made sure I did those exercises three times a day instead of once a day. The pain at first was horrible. I admit I cried on many occasions but it was what it was. I had heard the horrible stories of patients who did not rehab correctly or at all and some had died from blood clots. I was motivated."

Bennie's story was a little different. Initially, Bennie had a prescription for a home health nurse to come in and help her with the exercises she had been doing in the hospital.

She adds, "I argued for physical therapy and finally did get a prescription for additional therapy. He gave me a prescription for three weeks. Then my physical therapist recommended two to four additional weeks."

Bennie had some trouble with her leg feeling like it would give out. Her physical therapy lasted a little longer because of that. Her doctor advised her to use her walker as a precaution against falling when she went outside.

On the other side of the argument Joel, who is a physician's assistant with my surgeon, has this to say about prescribing physical therapy.

"I recommend all total knee patients do physical therapy in the hospital throughout their hospital stay and for 4 weeks after dismissal from the hospital. Some patients will require continued physical therapy based on their individual situation. Other patients elect to manage their own home rehabilitation due to cost, travel distance to the therapist, lack of a driver to physical therapy, or fear of outpatient physical therapy. I believe involvement of the physical therapy team in a total knee arthroplasty is one of the keys to a successful outcome and a pleased patient."

To Joel's comments, I can only add, Amen. I believe physical therapy is an important part of recovery. While we knee replacement patients were in the gym together we could compare notes, encourage each other, pick the therapists brains, and laugh or cry when needed.

Scott told a story of a man who, thinking he was tough, walked out of the hospital on his own steam and thought he could deal with recovery all on his own. The story ended with the man limping into physical therapy two weeks later. I don't know how accurate that story is. I do know that while I was in physical therapy several people who had not followed through with their prescribed therapy following injuries came into the gym. They came back because they had not been able to get full function back on their own.

There is a window of opportunity to get the joint moving again and to gain flexibility. Most people will tend to be stuck with whatever flexibility they have after four to six months. That does not leave a lot of time to wait.

Scott warned of the risk of the joint freezing up. I mentioned that possibility earlier. He had worked with patients who had a joint lock up and they had to go back into surgery and have the joint bent while they were under sedation. I would not want to wake up after that experience. Scott said it is not a bad as it sounds, but still....

Following my first knee operation I went into physical therapy after two weeks, the day after I had my staples removed. I was still using the walker. The walker was, by then, a crutch I unconsciously used to avoid putting my full weight on the operated leg. When I had the second knee replaced, six months after the first, the walker was gone by the end of the first week, and I was using a cane.

The problem with the walker, at least for me, was the tendency to lean on the thing and end up walking humped over it. The problem with crutches, which I used in an earlier unrelated surgery on my right knee, is that they are clumsy and like to fall on the floor when you are not looking. Whether you are using a walker to help your balance early in recovery as did most of the recipients I talked to, or crutches, the goal is to stop using any, excuse the pun, "crutch," and get back on your own two feet. With a broken leg the crutch or walker should take some of the weight while the bone heals. With a joint replacement the idea is to walk on the joint as soon as your doctor lets you so the joint can get stronger.

If you were using a cane or walker before the surgery, you might have to continue using it. I do suggest, if you have been using a walker or cane, to keep in mind the idea that the knee replacement might allow you to again walk without help. That is something for you and your doctor to decide.

Even when I quit using the walker and cane, I found my balance was a little off. When I stood, I had to make sure my feet were under me before setting off walking. I had a problem with balance throughout my recovery. The problem was noticeable enough that Scott commented on it. I always have listed a little to port. In my youth, every time I tried to water-ski I would plop over on my left side. I probably had a little more trouble with balance than a lot of my comrades in rehab.

It doesn't really seem to matter whether you start physical therapy before or after getting the staples out. I liked not having the staples pulling on my skin as I did my exercises. Some recipients I met started physical therapy before having their staples removed and did just fine.

When you do go in wear something loose and some shorts underneath. You will have to get down to shorts so the therapists can see what is going on and do what they need to. I also wore slip off shoes to make it easier to get them on and off when I had to work on a training table.

The general pattern of treatment, used by the facility where Scott works, is to start with comfort by reducing swelling and managing pain. Then the emphasis shifts to range of motion. The first range of motion goal is extension - how much can the person straighten their leg? When the patient can extend their leg fully, the goal shifts to flexion - how much can the person bend their leg? There is always an underlying goal of quad control and basic strength. Toward the end of therapy there is more focus on activities of daily living, (getting in and out of chairs, going up and down steps, getting into a car, dressing, getting to the bathroom), all the things a patient will want to be able to do after they are released from therapy.

The physical therapy sessions, when I started, were about an hour long. By the time I was finishing up, the sessions had stretched to an hour and a half. At first most of the time and energy focused on repair of the damage done by the surgery.

I was expecting a repeat of the type of exercises I had been doing at the hospital and at home after my release. Instead, the sessions started in a private room with an examining table and a machine with a bunch of buttons on it and a fistful of electric leads coming out of it. Scott proceeded to stick wires on my leg above and below the knee. He said he was going to give me the "Russian treatment." I got more than a little nervous when he paired the word Russian with electricity.

Actually, the "Russian" sends a small current through the knee joint and helps the fluid around your knee, which is responsible for the swelling, move off to another location and get absorbed. All I had to do was wait for the weird tingly feeling of the current to start and then try to force my knee down through the bed until the current and tingling stopped ten seconds later. After ten seconds of rest another round started. That went on for twenty minutes. It was harder to get the muscle going than I thought it would be. When I was done, Scott iced the knee for a while and sent me home.

I was surprised at all the attention on getting the leg straight. Scott explained that if a patient does not get their leg straight, standing for any length of time will be very hard. Try standing for fifteen minutes with your leg slightly bent and see how long it is before you get uncomfortable. Most knee recipients find their operated leg gets its full extension in about two weeks. If you could straighten your leg all the way before the surgery you will probably be able to straighten it fully with the new knee.

The procedure for getting the knee to fully extend is straightforward if a little uncomfortable. You have probably already done the initial exercise, called the "quad set". This is the exercise where you sit or lie on a table and try to contract your quadriceps as if you were driving your knee down so you leg is flat on the table. The electric stimulation machine helps the quads wake up from the trauma of being cut during surgery. This time the electrodes go above the knee to focus on the quadriceps. The stimulation, like in the Russian, is intense but it does not hurt.

The other exercise used to straighten the leg is to prop the heel on a can wrapped in a towel for a minute or two. This passive exercise was surprisingly uncomfortable even though I was doing nothing but lying on the table. Those two exercises started each of the physical therapy session for the first three weeks.

The next goal of therapy is the expected one of getting the operated knee to bend. Some knee recipients have had limited flexibility for years. The limits come from muscles and tendons shrinking when they are not used. A knee recipient who was previously limited may not get back all of the flexibility they lost, though many do regain more than they had before having the knee replaced. This is a much more complicated process than straightening the leg. There are a lot more exercises and steps to take. Many of the initial exercises are the same ones you are familiar with from the hospital. As you get stronger, your therapist will introduce you to other exercises which are not a part of the at home routine.

None of the exercises are terribly complex. Most are hard when the patient first tries to do them and get easier as with practice. All of the exercises are a necessary part of recovery. Each one focuses on flexibility, strength, or balance.

Watch it though. Physical therapists are sneaky. They start to add more repetition and more weight when they think their charge is having too easy a time with the exercises. I do jest. The extra reps and weight help the person get stronger. Accusing the therapists of making it hard on purpose was a way for those of us in rehab to lighten the mood. Of course, whining and complaining didn't do any good.

No matter which physical therapy gym you attend you will encounter the "Nu-Step" machine. There is no generic name for this device, according to Scott, as the company has the patent on this "torture device." You likely will not face the machine during the first week or even the second since the early sessions focus more on extension. When the emphasis of physical therapy changes to flexion, that is bending the knee, you will meet the Nu-Step.

The device looks like a cross between a reclining bicycle and a stair climber. The patient sits on a seat with their legs extended to two pedals. The patient alternately presses one pedal and then the other, like they were using a stair climbing machine. When the patient extends one leg to push the pedal away from their body, the other pedal comes back toward the body, flexing the knee.

When the patient can easily push the pedal forward to its limits there is a nice solid, satisfying clunk as the pedal hits a stop. When I first heard the clunk I was hoping that was it for the Nu-Step. Unfortunately, there is an adjustment which moves the seat closer to the pedals which increases the amount the knee flexes each time the opposite pedal is pushed forward by the good leg.

I gave the machine the most curses for being hard, and the most praise for allowing me to see progress as the weeks passed. After I met the Nu-Step, my trainer made it the first exercise of each session. I must say I liked the machine in spite of my love-hate relationship because I could push myself and measure progress by how close the seat was to the pedals.

Motivation is a key in recovery. Several people n the gym said they loved the Nu-Step. I couldn't understand why until I realized it would be easy to go through the motions while not pushing hard. Maybe some of those who claimed to love the machine were "dogging it" on the Nu-Step to avoid the other exercises where the therapist could keep closer watch.

Another focus of therapy is gait training. I had to work hard to get rid of the nasty limp I developed over the years of dealing with the pain of my bad knees. After surgery I continued to drag the operated leg forward without bending the knee, thus walking stiff legged. It hurt less than bending the knee when I walked. The limp caused by not bending the knee was different than the one I had had for years. But it was still a limp. Scott made me walk down the hall each session and made frequent corrections of my bad habits. After several months I could consistently walk with a smooth, normal gait and not think about what I was doing at each step

Scott spent a lot of time drilling me on the proper gait: lift the foot of the operated leg, bend the knee, pull the leg forward with the quadriceps, straighten the knee and set the heel down. Practicing hard at this point in recovery makes it much easier later.

I found it was easier to keep a proper gait going when I was out for a longer walk, than when I was schlepping around in the kitchen.

While I was in physical therapy, I continued doing the exercises my surgeon had me doing before surgery. These are the same ones the hospital physical therapists started me on following surgery. Doing those exercises three times a day was a good supplement to the three times a week physical therapy sessions. Think of these exercises as homework.

I asked Scott if there are different standards for flexion based on the age of the knee recipient. He said the goal he sets is 120° for everyone, though he tends to push the younger and more active clients to be more functional. The older and less active clients often pay more attention to eliminating pain than regaining a high level of functionality. The older client is often not as concerned with being able to get down on the floor and up again.

Another aspect of how motivated the knee recipient is may have to do with the aging process. I recognize I am slowing down, but am not willing to give up activities because I am "old." I can see how a person who sees his or her self as old could develop the attitude that they are stiff just because they are old. I was surprised to find in one study I ran across that the average range of motion for people who have not had replacement surgery was 132°. There was only a 3° difference between the younger age group starting at age 25, and the oldest group which reached up to age 74. (Physical Therapy, Sep. 1, 1991, Kathryn Roach, "Normal hip and knee ROM: the relationship to age.")

NINE

"I THINK I'LL LIVE"

Most knee replacement recipients come to the awareness about three weeks into recovery that there might be an end to the pain after all. The fiery pain usually starts to ease up some in week three and slowly decreases over the next few months. It feels good to have some relief from the fierce pain that has been present since surgery. When this pain starts easing up most of the recipients started believing that recovery was actually happening.

Everyone who is taking the narcotic pain killers will have to talk to their doctor to decide how long to continue the medications. The reports I have heard range from one to six weeks.

I was sent home with a prescription for 30 tablets, and the instructions to take up to four a day. The prescription had one refill. I started tapering off the tablets after being home a few days and took the last one sometime in the third week I was home. I did not refill the

94

prescription. From then on I relied on over the counter pain meds. I am not a pill taker, so getting off the narcotics sooner rather than later fit my philosophy that any pain I was experiencing, after the fierce pain that followed surgery had passed, was a guide to how hard I was pushing myself. One nurse who had a bilateral replacement was just starting to wean off the narcotics after four weeks.

Standing and walking still caused a strong sense of pressure and pain. I felt the knee with every step.

You may also begin to feel that the pain is moving around from spot to spot around your knee. I'm not sure why the pain seems to move around in the joint, but it is a common experience. My belief is that, as the swelling goes out of one spot and that spot stops hurting, you become aware of some other spot that still has swelling and pain. The pain of surgery masked these other pains, because the pain of the surgery itself was so great. As long as these traveling pains do not get worse or severe you can take the moving pains as part of healing.

At one point it felt like the surgeon had beaten my shin with a hammer. I had a terrible pain in my shin whenever I had been sitting for a while and stood up. The leg felt like it would give out any moment. I had to hobble and steady myself for ten or fifteen steps before the pain eased up and I could walk without hobbling. I asked Joel about it and he said blood can pool in that area during surgery and it will hurt until the body clears away all the blood in the area. I have not looked at a tape of my operation, so I can't prove my doctor did not beat my leg with a hammer. Joel seems like an honest person, and my surgeon does not seem like the type to abuse a patient so I will take their word for it.

I adopted an attitude of patience and as time went on all the little and big "owies" went away. It does take a long time though, so don't get impatient. You are less than a month into recovery and there is still quite a bit of swelling in the knee. My therapist said it would take three months for all the swelling to clear out of the joint.

It started to be easier to get in and out of the car. Also, the pain of the bumps in the road lessened. After several weeks of physical therapy I could bend my knee enough to squeeze my toes in and out of the car door without having to lay down the seat back or move the seat all the way to the rear. That was a red letter day.

You may be able to, with some effort, lift your operated leg straight over the edge of the tub and step in. This became another daily exercise. Each day I would lift my operated leg as high as I could. At first it barely edged past the lip of the tub. As I kept practicing, my toes cleared the tub lip by a little more each day or so. A trick that helps is to flex your foot up as you lift the leg. If you just concentrate on lifting the leg the foot will droop down and get in the way. The foot drop goes away as you get stronger.

There are still plenty of naps. Your body needs a lot of time to heal after the large trauma of knee replacement surgery. Whether you rest in your bed or in a lounge chair, you will often sit down to read or watch TV and wake up a few hours later. My advice is to enjoy the naps and not think you should be more awake.

You should continue with the ice packs and keep your leg elevated when you are resting.

Getting back into the drivers seat of your car depends on two things. One factor is that you are no longer taking the narcotic pain medication. The narcotics slow a person's reflexes and may make him or her feel drowsy. The other thing that will keep you out of the driver's seat is simply not being able to bend the knee enough, or your leg may not be strong enough to work the pedals. Most of the knee recipients I talked to were driving between three and six weeks. I was able to get in the driver's seat and take myself to physical therapy after three weeks. My wife was glad not to have to take any more time off work to take me to the gym, so she didn't mind me driving again.

Gisele said it was hard for her to bend her knee enough to easily move her foot from the gas to the brake. It was more than three weeks before she could drive.

If your right knee is the one which was replaced you will feel strange sensations and perhaps a little pain in the knee when you lift it from the gas to the brake and back again, even though the leg is strong enough to do the work of braking and accelerating. I was careful when I first started driving. I felt unsure of myself and was a little slow moving my leg from the gas to the brake.

If your operated leg is the left one, you may be in the driver's seat sooner. All you have to do is be able to drag it into the car.

Though you may be able to drive the knee will still respond to every bump in the road.

The fact that I was able to drive did not inspire me to go out and run around town. I only drove to physical therapy and home. When I was done I wanted nothing more than to take a nap.

My original foolish plan was to go back to work after two weeks. My work consists of sitting and listening to people. It seemed like it would be simple to go sit at my office instead of in my recliner. At the end of the first month I was still struggling to stay awake through the day. Give yourself plenty of time to heal before trying work. Also remember that we are older than we were when we might have broken an arm as a child and we heal slower. There are some things that do not change.

PART THREE:

USE IT

THE NEXT FIVE MONTHS

Sometime after the first month has passed the new knee owner will feel well enough to start thinking of doing more than going to physical therapy, eating, watching TV, and sleeping. From now until the six month mark of recovery the focus is on getting more confident and trusting the knee. Physical therapy puts more emphasis on the owner's ability to walk smoothly, handle stairs, and get back to what used to be normal activities.

The tricks focus more toward the owner using the new knee and getting back into the old routine, without the pain and limping of course. The question of, "When is this ever going to end?" will rear its head from time to time.

TEN

"I'M GOING STIR CRAZY"

The watchword for the second month is – "use it". This is a time when a lot of healing occurs, but the knee is still functioning well below full capacity.

Physical therapy continues. The good news is your muscles are getting stronger and you can have more confidence that you are able to move around safely. The exercises at home and in the gym start to be less of an agony and more of a workout.

One day, perhaps when you wake up in the morning, you become aware that you are not thinking about the new knee. This pleasant experience lasts but a moment at first, though it is a hopeful moment. For the next several months the joint will not let you forget it for very long. It will stiffen up, give you weird sensations, and ache. Even with a warning like you've just read, you can start to believe it will get better.

At first the trick of sitting and standing from a straight chair is not pretty and involves a lot of leaning forward and grunting when sitting down and getting up. The first time I asked my operated leg to work that hard the muscles protested I had to use my hands to push off the chair or grab the edge of the table, whichever was closest, to pull myself up. Each week the push was a little less, but it was there. Using my hands helped take the strain off the knee. Even with this new trick it is hard to sit for long. The knee stiffened up quickly and I had to stretch it often. But the knee took the strain and I gave a big sigh when my bottom was finally in the chair seat. In spite of the downside of sitting in a straight chair it is nice to be able to sit at the table long enough to finish a meal. Eating at the table is an activity that just feels normal.

It is a relief the first day you are able to sit in a chair with your bottom all the way on the chair and the knee bent enough that the hamstring is not jammed into the edge of the chair seat.

Crossing your legs is not in the cards as it hurts too much.

I started going back to church about this time. One thing to look for when you start going to church, or to any event with aisle seating, is an aisle seat. Your knee will not let you be comfortable for more than a few minutes if you cannot stretch it frequently. I always tried to sit on the aisle so I could stretch my leg out in the aisle. Very few venues have leg room to really stretch out.

A milestone is when you can sit on the edge of the bed and lift the operated leg enough to just barely get the knee bent enough to put on socks and shoes. Putting on your socks and shoes sounds easy but is definitely hard when the joint does not want to bend and there is pain when you lift the leg. For the first few weeks I did this trick it felt like heel slides which, as you will learn, hurt when you get close to the maximum you can flex your knee.

During the second month going up and down steps gets a little easier though you will still be "one stepping" it until you have had a chance to practice with your therapist and get approval.

Learning to "two step" on stairs starts in physical therapy when you have gained some flexibility, strength and balance. At first the trainer directs the person to practice stepping onto and back off of a low stool. The exercise is simple. Lift the foot of the operated leg onto a stool and push with the operated leg to raise the body, and then step up with the good leg. You complete the exercise by stepping back down with first the good then the operated leg. You will fee the normal pain/discomfort you feel with any of your exercises. Those who have had both knees done at the same time just have to alternate which leg they use to lift their weight.

When you are stronger at this exercise your therapist will take you out to a real flight of stairs for practice. Climbing stairs at this point is a deliberate, one leg at a time affair. Being human the temptation is to want to sort of hop with the good leg to give yourself a boost. Don't let your therapist catch you doing it. Lift the operated leg up to the next step then push with the operated leg to lift your weight, just as you were doing in the gym. Don't use the handrail to pull yourself up. Don't swing your operated leg to the side to clear the step. The trick of lifting the toes which you may have used to step into the shower, will help you lift your leg straight up and not out to the side.

The object is to stand straight lift your operated knee to the next step by bending the knee and lift your weight with each leg in turn. Climbing stairs so deliberately will "feel" funny. Just keep it up. Like getting back to a normal walking gait, it is one of those things you have to relearn after years of cheating because of the old pain.

The trick of "two stepping" down steps comes a week or so after you start going up the stairs. You start practicing in the physical therapy gym by stepping onto the same low stool you used when you were practicing going up. Instead of stepping back off the stool, you now step forward off of it. The good leg leads and the quadriceps muscle of your operated leg lowers your weight to the ground.

Recipients have a tendency to protect the muscle by letting their weight "fall" off the stool and using the leading good leg to catch it. Cheating will hurt less initially but will not strengthen the muscles and eventually be able to go easily down stairs. At first, when you are stepping down it feels as if the leg will buckle when you are lowering your weight with it. The knee pulls and pains as you step down. Be patient, it takes time before you feel comfortable going down stairs. When you are ready your therapist will let you graduate to the stairs at the clinic.

The stairs you practice on at the hospital or therapist's office may be wider and shallower than the ones you will have to manage at home. The stairs at my house are narrow and my foot does not fit all the way onto the tread. It's kind of like "hanging ten" on a surfboard. For a long time I had to turn my body at an angle so my foot would fit well enough that I felt stable. Because of the narrow tread I had to hold on to the handrail at home for a few weeks until I felt steadier.

* * *

The End of Physical Therapy

I felt like going up and down stairs was sort of a final exam for therapy. If you can bend the knee enough to go up and down stairs you will be able to accomplish most of the daily tasks you will need to do.

Toward the end of therapy you will have almost as much range of motion in your knee as you are going to have. The full range of motion for a new, original equipment knee is about150°. That's the reason youngsters can sit back on their heels without a thought. By the time most of us have reached the age when we need new knees we will have a range of motion between 130° and 140°.

My therapist says he targets for 120°of flexion no matter what the age of the client. Scarring from the surgery limits most people's post recovery range of motion by five or ten degrees.

A common belief is that range of motion is reduced as a function of getting older. That does not seem to be the case. Many older individuals remain flexible. The idea that we automatically get less flexible as we get older may be more of a function of whether we keep moving or sit down. If you can attain a range of motion of 120° you will have plenty of flexibility to sit and stand easily from a chair, climb stairs, get in and out of cars, and lift your foot onto a chair to tie your shoe. It is enough to climb a ladder, though your doctor many not recommend the latter activity due to the risk of damaging the knee if you should fall. It is enough to get onto the floor to play with the grandkids and get up again.

My therapist released me after my first replacement with a flexion score of 116°. When I left therapy for the left knee, six months later, the right knee was bending at 126 degrees. I had gained almost 10 degrees of flexion after therapy simply by using the knee.

My therapist, Scott, said that he could tell when a knee locks up and cannot go any further. He never told me that my knee was as far as it would go. I did experience going to the limit one time when I stepped off the edge of a porch about three feet high. I can tell you it hurts to be at maximum flexion that way. One younger patient said when she left physical therapy she was able to get her knee to bend to 130° after three months. That was Gisele who had some extra time in therapy due to her knee being exceptionally tight.

In the first two months of recovery most of my attention had been on the daily exercises, taking short walks and looking forward to the Monday, Wednesday and Friday morning physical therapy sessions. I enjoyed spending time with the staff who acted as cheerleaders, and the other patients who had undergone the experience of having a joint replaced. I was able to tell myself while I was still going to the physical therapy gym that I was not yet healed. When those three times a week sessions ended I had to start thinking of what I was going to do from that point on.

One of my favorite exercises before the operation was bike riding. It was something I could do without hurting my bad knees. While I was still in physical therapy I asked to try the stationary bike. I was worried I might not be able to ride with the new knee. The fact that I could, with difficulty, get the pedals on the stationary bike to go around, gave me confidence that I would be able to get back on two wheels. If you try the stationary bike, you will find that, for some reason, it is easier to turn the pedals backward rather than forward.

Finishing therapy is a great morale booster. I remember standing by the elevator after my last session feeling light and airy because I had just successfully completed therapy. The nostalgia for the people I had worked with came later. Graduating, however, does not mean that everything is all right. There is a long way to go to feel comfortable letting the artificial knee do its job.

***

The swelling in your knee may be down enough that it is not necessary to have the ice pack on the joint 24/7. I was relieved when I didn't have to go to the refrigerator five times a day to change it out. And it was nice to be able to sleep without fighting with an ice bag. I do recommend putting ice on the knee for an hour after working out, doing your home exercises, or going for a longer walk. The interior of your knee still has some swelling even if you can now see your knee dimples.

When I could see my knee dimples, I started leaving the ice pack off at night. What a relief. One lady said her physical therapist told her one day, "I love your wrinkles." She was somewhat offended until the therapist said it was nice that the swelling had gone down enough for the wrinkles to show.

At the end of two months I was glad to be into some kind of normal sleep pattern. It was a great day when I could roll over on my stomach for a few minutes. There was a weird sensation on the front of the knee as it pressed on the bed. It was not painful and faded over a few weeks. The best part of lying on my stomach was not having the pressure of being on my back.

One recipient listed sleeping as the biggest frustration. He said he had great difficulty sleeping because of the pain. The pills helped some but he had this deep down feeling that it still hurt. It was months before he could sleep for any length of time.

For the first month lying on my side had been impossible because the weight of the good leg lying on the operated leg made the joint hurt. I tried to lie on the other side with the operated leg on top. That hurt too. I tried to stretch the leg out but that hurt just as much as having it bent. I was stuck on my back.

When I was finally able to lie on my side it was only a few minutes before my leg started hurting. Even though I could not stay on my side for long, it felt good to have the pressure off my back. A small pillow between my legs, just above the knees, helped ease the pressure a little and let me stay on my side longer.

Unfortunately, I was not able to stay on my side long enough to fall asleep. Each night it seemed I got a few more minutes of relief. And then one night I fell asleep on my side. The sleep only lasted for an hour or so before the ache in my leg woke me up and I had to shift onto my back. After a few more weeks I could sleep on my side for several hours, before I had to turn onto my back.

Another side sleeper is still using a pillow between her knees after nine months. She isn't complaining since she is able to sleep through the night.

ELEVEN

A SEMBLANCE OF NORMAL

Going into the third month of recovery, if you are like most recipients, your knee will feel better, much of the swelling and pain is gone and you have more energy, and are eager to be more active. Over the next three months, the second quarter of the year following your surgery, you will feel like doing more of the activities you were hoping the knee replacement would allow you to do. Feel free to do as much as you can without undue strain. Though you are feeling better, you are still not up to full speed. Allow plenty of time for rest and don't expect to be able to do everything you could before your knee, or knees, went bad – not yet anyway.

I began to think I might actually want to do something more than take short walks, read and watch television. In short I was going stir-crazy. I wanted to do more than take short walks in my sweats, with my wife along for moral support. Now I wanted to get up and go out on my own. I wanted to go downtown, and to the grocery store. It was time to return to life.

Though the knee feels better most of the time, it still gives problems. I found it hard not to favor the operated leg. I found myself stiff-legging it rather than bending the knee. I favored the leg when I stood or sat. There were aches and pains when I walked a lot. The aches and pains are a regular part of the day, but you can see them as a normal part of healing.

I stopped doing the home exercises when I stopped going to physical therapy. I asked for a list of exercises to do for follow-up, but the list I received was the same list of exercises I had been doing since before going in for the surgery. I admit I was pretty bored with those exercises. It had been routine to do the three sets of ten for each exercise, then get up and do what I had planned for the day. Looking back, if I had continued with any of the exercises it would have been the heel slides, pulling the foot along a flat surface with a towel under the heel to draw the leg up to the body and flex the knee. That one exercise focuses specifically on flexion in the knee.

When I talked to my therapist some months after I was done with therapy, he said he recommended that the patient keep doing the exercises. He said it was especially important for the patient to continue with those strengthening and flexibility exercises if he or she was not active. He was right. If the owner of the new knee is not active he or she could lose strength and flexibility.

Progress for the next several months consists in consolidating the improvements gained in therapy. I spent a lot of time working on walking with a natural gait; lift the leg, pull it through, straighten it up and set it down. There was a strong tendency to "stiff leg" it by pulling the leg forward without bending the knee. I thank my wife for pointing it out to me more than a few times.

This is a good time to expand your walks, perhaps from down the street to around the block. I began to dress in more than sweats and socks. Expanding walks brings a new set of discomforts. When the knee is used more you will get some soreness and stiffness. You may have muscle cramps in your legs and feet, as you work out the kinks.

Some recipients experience pain in their feet and ankles. The surgery may straighten your leg or even change its length, remember a plastic disk now fills the space of lost cartilage, enough that the other parts of your leg have to get used to the change. When I started walking more I noticed pain in my feet and ankles. I had been bowlegged all my life and the other parts of my legs had to get used to the fact that my legs were now straight.

One lady, who had been quite bowlegged, said that her shoes no longer felt right and she had to get new shoes for walking. She figured out that while she had been so bowlegged she had worn her shoes in a way that no longer fit her walking gait. The solution was easy for her; buy some new walking shoes.

Another said she spent more time in physical therapy getting ultrasound for an irritated Iliotibial band (A length of tendon that runs from the hip to the knee) than on flexibility exercises. She did say that she had had the syndrome before the operation.

Stretching your walk can have some unexpected benefits. When my walks extended around the block I started passing a friend's house. Usually, he was at work, but one day he was out working in the yard. My friend noticed me about a half-block from his house. He stopped his yard work and leaned on his lawn mower. I was still some way away when he called out, "Hey. Dave! Your surgery must have worked. I haven't seen you walk so straight in years." I hadn't really thought about it but my surgeon had made my bowlegs straight. Not only was I not limping I was walking straight up.

How far should you walk? The only answer I can give is to go as far as you can without overdoing it. At first, going around the block was pushing it. Half-way around the block, I could feel the tiredness. By the time I got home, I was ready to sit down for a while and put some ice on my knee. I was usually feeling rested after another hour. That seems like a long rest for a short walk. You are still recovering so plan on a longer recovery time than you might like.

In the old days, I was one of those people who ran road races – my status was participant. Paula is the one who has a drawer full of medals – I learned that it takes two weeks for the body to adjust to a new level of exertion. Using that rule you should stay at a given distance for two weeks before trying to increase the distance – slowly.

Though most of the pain of surgery is gone, and the swelling is mostly out of the knee, there remains a sensation of pressure/pulling with each step and every time the knee is bent. It isn't quite pain, but the sensation is noticeable. My best description is that sometimes it feels like little jolts of electricity. One person described it as feeling like a bunch of bees buzzing around inside the knee.

When the swelling seemed to be out of the knee, I noticed that the joint always seemed to be warm. I wondered if that was something that would last forever. It did not. I suspect that the warmth was from residual swelling deep inside. I also worried that the knees might get cold in the winter. That did not happen. I cannot remember the knees feeling cold because of the metal in them

The knee still gives a lot of signals it is not completely healed. Standing on it for more than 15 minutes causes the knee to stiffen and ache. When you start to walk the knee may hurt for the first half dozen steps. The knee also tends to hurt during the act of sitting down. There are a lot of moments during the day when the knee announces its presence. But the pain is now manageable. The biggest danger for the owner is to say it hurts too much and to stop moving the joint. During this "Use It" period the most important issue is to keep the joint moving. In time all of these aches and pains will go away.

There is still something like pain when walking. Pain is probably not the best word. Maybe the best way to describe the feeling is that it is more like a bruise. Most of us remember having a big bruise that hurts a bit each time we take a step, but the pain is not so bad that we limp or that it gets worse as the day goes on. I finally came up with the term "residual discomfort" to describe the fact that you can still tell your knee is not original equipment, but it works fine to get you around.

As my knee healed I began to wonder about a patch of skin, about six inches across, below the knee and toward the outside that felt funny when I touched it. It was not quite numb but definitely did not feel normal.

During the operation the surgeon had to cut the intrapattellar branch of the saphenous nerve. The nerve is small and superficial, and is cut to expose the knee so the components of the replacement can be properly installed. The result of cutting the nerve is that the small circle of skin goes numb. Rather than being totally numb area just feels weird. In normal day to day activities the sensation fades into the background. It is there if you rub on it, or if someone else touches the spot. You also feel it when you kneel down on the knee. Otherwise you will lose track of the spot.

Joel said the surrounding nerves innervate (invade) the area over six to twelve months. Some people feel sensitivity to touch or a burning sensation as a result. I had worried that jeans or other rough fabric might cause a problem, but clothing does not cause any unusual sensations in the area. I have noticed, now that I have had my knees for over a year, that there are times when I feel a slight burning sensation. The sensation is minor and does not cause problems.

You might try working on the trick of standing up when putting on your pants if you feel up to it and were able to manage the task before surgery. When I started working on this feat, it was a test of my balance and to force myself to bend my knee as far as it would go. Holding the waistband of a pair of drawers or pants, and balancing at the same time may be a challenge. I had a tendency to fall out of balance. It was hard to bend over and at the same time lift my leg enough to get my toes in the hole.

I suggest staying near a solid object so you can catch yourself on those times you lose your balance. I liked to stand by the bed so I could just plop down if I needed to. I could also cheat by leaning against the bed for balance. More than a few times I had to drop whatever I was trying to get into and set my foot down to keep from taking a tumble. It is better to try again than to fall. When I was much younger I didn't mind falling. I knew how to do a pratfall. With age comes wisdom, or at least caution. On days when I didn't feel as confident I just sat on the edge of the bed and put my feet through the holes.

You may find yourself feeling pretty good and staying up all day without taking long naps, though your energy levels are not yet up to full charge. Be aware you don't have the energy to do everything you did before the surgery. I spent a lot of time watching TV and telling myself I needed to get started on things. I didn't get started. Just getting the things necessary to get through the day wore me out. Though you might have enough energy left to help a little with the cooking and dish washing.

I was back at work by the start of the third month. I had thought I could start back after two weeks and then changed it to a month. That didn't work out even though my work is not labor intensive. I sit in a chair and listen to people talk about their troubles. I found it hard to concentrate for the hour an appointment lasts. My knee got stiff and sore and I was constantly changing its position. I couldn't cross my legs, either one, without it hurting. I spent a lot of the days trying to ignore the ache in my leg. I got the work done but was happy to go home at the end of a short day.

Most knee recipients start getting back to work slowly, with half days or several days a week off. One nurse who had both knees done at once, and whose job kept her on her feet all day, was twelve weeks post surgery and thinking about going back to work part time. Another man in the same age group was planning to start back part time at his retail job two months after surgery. I did meet a man, in his mid fifties, who said he went back to work in a factory in two weeks. I found it hard to believe, but there are some people who are a lot tougher than I am.

At night I was tired enough to sleep because I was tired and not because of exhaustion. I was able to mostly sleep through the night without the knee waking me up every hour.

I learned the trick of sitting and standing from a straight-back chair without pushing off with my hands. I had been sticking my operated leg out in front – trick number two – and lowering my self into the chair with my good leg while holding on to a table or supporting myself on the chair arms or seat. Now I needed to figure out how to sit down using just my legs.

The technique is not complicated. Get your feet level with each other and your legs just touching the front of the chair seat, then lower your body –sounds easy. The trick is that you have to lean much farther forward than you would think, to balance the fact that your legs are not nearly as strong as they were before the surgery, in spite of the physical therapy you have done. And you have to lower yourself slowly and smoothly, and not just plop down.

There is nothing complicated abut standing from a chair, but you will probably have to lean forward more than you did before the surgery. When getting up it is cheating to bounce up to give your self a boost.

Here is another trick you can try to get the knee to bend further. While sitting at table or in church, pull the lower leg back as far as possible using its own strength, then hook your ankle with your other foot and pull back a little more. Hold it in that position until it starts to be more uncomfortable than you want to deal with. The practice will help the knee get more flexible and useful.

TWELVE

THE TRICKS ARE NEARLY ALL LEARNED
(It's time to get out and move it.)

By the beginning of the fourth month following surgery the majority of recipients have learned most of the tricks they will need to get through their days. You can use the knee, though it still reminds you frequently of the trauma to muscle and bone. This is frustrating because recovery has seemed to last forever, and you might think the pain should all be gone. Be patient. It will be some while before you forget, most of the time, that you have an artificial knee. In the meantime, remember what it felt like to use the knee before your surgery. One knee recipient put it well when she said, "I am so far ahead of where I was before the surgery. I should have done this long ago."

I started sleeping through the night. The length of time I could sleep on my side gradually increased through the month until I was sleeping in my old normal pattern of spending the night on my side. Getting back to my old ritual was a big improvement and made for better rest. If you are a stomach or back sleeper you may already be sleeping through the night.

I even woke up many mornings thinking about something other than the knee, though I became aware of the knee as soon as I stood up. The joint was stiff and a little "owie." I was wobbly for the first few steps in the morning. But I was far enough along in recovery I could believe the joint was healing just fine and go on with the day.

On the days when I overused the new knee it got a little sore. The soreness was mostly in the muscles and went away with a night's rest. The wonderful part was that the overuse did cause me to limp or cause the kind of pain that was present before the surgery.

I was eager to get back on my bike saddle. My riding was not the long distance type, but nice thirty-minute rides around town or on the local bike paths. When I finally got back on my bike in the real world I had to raise the seat up as high as it would go and still reach the pedals. I had a hard time getting my knee to bend enough so I could get the pedals all the way around. The first few cranks of the pedals were always hard and hurt a little, but the knee loosened up quickly. When my knee was comfortable with the highest seat position, I lowered the seat a half inch and repeated the process. After a month of lowering my seat at half inch increments, I was sitting so low I could barely turn the pedals over. The lower the seat on a bicycle the harder it is to push the pedals because the more you bend your legs the less power you have to push the pedals.

When I couldn't lower the seat anymore and still turn the crank, I put the seat back where I had it before surgery and kept riding.

Bicycle riding is good exercise since it does not put a lot of stress on the knees. The most demanding part of riding is going uphill since it takes more work and puts more stress on your knees, not to mention your breathing. Shifting to a lower gear (moving the chain to a smaller sprocket) on hills reduces the load on the knees and breathing. If you are not familiar with downshifting, it will take only a few minutes of practice on level ground to locate those gears which make it possible to easily pedal up hills. If a hill gets too steep, it is not against the rules to get off and walk the bike to the top.

One lady with a double knee replacement was riding around the park about ten weeks after surgery and said it was much better for her than walking. At that time she was still walking with a stiff legged gait, though she said it was far better than before the replacements. I knew her before and she looked like she had been on horseback her whole life

Not everyone likes to ride around on a bike. An exercise bike may be a good substitute to get the knees moving without putting a lot of weight on the joint.

I do believe, though, that walking is a necessary exercise for everyone. Walking puts some weight on the joint, which is good. Bones get stronger when they have some stress on them every day.

There are two types of exercise which might be called aerobic and load bearing. Aerobic exercises build up the person's lungs and the ability to continue an activity for a long time. An exercise like bike riding has a large aerobic component. Turning the pedals is a repetitious activity that does not put a large amount of stress on the body. Programs like Jazzercise, Tai-Chi, and cycling are examples of exercises that are repetitious. Doing this type of exercise faster, makes us breathe harder and build up endurance but does not make us lift more each time the routine is done.

Load bearing exercises, on the other hand, focus on building up the muscles and strengthening the bones. The classic load bearing exercise is weight lifting. In weight lifting the object is to train the body's ability to lift heavier and heavier loads.

Walking combines both types of exercises. Unlike cycling where the only effort is to turn the pedals, in walking a person has to lift the weight of their own body with one leg and move the body forward with each step. That's the load bearing part of walking. The aerobic part of walking is that when a person walks faster they are building up their lungs. If they walk farther they are building up their endurance. Walking is an easily performed triple play of exercise.

At the end of three months I was walking up to a mile, and able to ride my bike for thirty minutes or so. The knee was still a little sore when I got done, and my muscles complained at the end of a mile. But I had not even been able to walk a mile before surgery without it wiping me out for the rest of the day, and part of the next.

The point of this chapter is that, though a knee recipient has learned all they need in order to get through their days in a few months, it is not enough. If the new knee owner wants to recover to his or her full potential, he or she needs to find a way to get active.

The most assertive statement anyone made about getting back to doing normal activities was the woman who had her surgery in early February and by the end of April was playing golf. She did confess that she was riding in a cart and that she was very protective of her knee. All I can say is, "You know how golfers are."

THIRTEEN

THREE MONTHS OF SLOW WORK
(Working Your Way Through the Second Quarter of Recovery)

Activities which are difficult but doable now will make the joint more functional in the long run. Using the joint makes it stronger and more useful. However, you need to remember that there is still a lot of healing to do. You are sort of like a ballplayer that has surgery and goes down to the minors for a year to recover before he or she can play at full strength.

It is pleasant to get feedback from family and friends on how good you are doing. Like with most changes, those around you will see that you have changed before you are comfortable with the skills you have regained during recovery.

As the pace of recovery slows there are few tricks yet to learn. Most of the emphasis is on getting back to using the knee normally. Don't rush it. From now on it is a matter of letting the slow process of recovery work.

You can still feel the knee when walking, though there is little if any pain. It is hard to describe just how it feels to walk. All the parts seem to work, yet everything seems to be just a little out of adjustment. Every step up and down a curb or stair takes a little bit more attention to do it smoothly. There are frequently times when you will need to make a slight adjustment to maintain balance. In short, nothing seems to flow as it used to. This is a bit frustrating, but is only a stage. The sensation of your muscles pulling and stretching when you walk continues to slowly diminish.

Any feeling that the knee is going to give out is most evident when going down stairs.

I still noticed a bit of limping or stiff-legging when I was moving around the house and was not taking full strides. There is just not enough room to get going at a steady pace, and getting a steady pace is necessary to stretch the muscles and keep the knee loose.

Pain is still noticeable when you have to stand for a long time. The knee gets stiff and starts to ache. The only remedy is to bend it to get the stiffness out, or to walk around to loosen the knee up. Even so, you can stand on it for an hour or more without a problem. I was pleased with this development since it meant I could get back to singing with the choir at Sunday services.

Even with all the lingering issues, this is a time period when confidence in walking increases dramatically. There are times, especially when your mind is on something else that you will be walking with a normal, natural gait and not be aware of it.

I tried to walk every day. Walking is always good exercise, and, when not overdone, helps keep the knee loose. Our joints are a bit like cars. Use them or they will rust up and do not move at all. One of my thoughts is that as we get older we do not push our bodies as far as they will go. I'm not talking extreme sports here just bending, stretching, and moving. Studies show that an older person, who begins an exercise program, even after being idle for years, becomes more mobile and has better balance.

If you were able, before the surgery, to step put of a car on one leg, now might be a good time to start up again. Before the fourth month the only way I could enter and exit a car was to swing both legs around, so my feet were on the ground, and then stand up using the door for leverage and balance. Getting in and out by putting one foot outside the car and using only that one leg to step out and stand up may seem a daunting task. For several months you have probably swiveled out of the car, just as I did, so neither leg carried your full weight.

To start getting both of your legs strong enough to carry all of your body weight go ahead and use the door to help lever yourself up. The trick is not complicated, just set one leg out on the ground, lean into it and push to stand. As with each of the new tricks following surgery this one is hard at first and there may be twinges of pain. On the other hand the practice will strengthen your legs and give back a skill which gives you more freedom of movement.

There may come a day when you can lift your foot up onto a chair to tie your shoe more easily. The simple act involves flexibility as well as balance. Lifting your foot onto a chair puts you in position for another informal exercise to flex the knee as far as it will go. Leave you foot flat on the chair and push your body forward. This will cause the knee to flex more than when you are just walking or sitting. If you could not put your foot up on a chair before your surgery, you might try this exercise on a lower surface such as a step stool.

Here is a caution. It is easier to step up on a chair than to step down. I don't know why this is but it is true. It may be something to do with how the quad works or stretches more when stepping up than stepping down. I once found myself stranded when I stepped up onto a chair to find something in a closet and had to call Paula to lend me a hand to get down. Stepping down tall steps is still an issue.

By the end of six months you may be able to walk for several miles at a time. If you were in fairly good shape before surgery, this should not be a stretch. I had my second surgery in the middle of October. At the end of March, with two new knees, Paula and I flew to Chicago for a few days. This was only five and a half months after I got my second new knee. Paula was attending a conference for her work, and I was tagging along for company. We stayed in a downtown hotel, and, as is our custom, did not rent a car.

I was delighted that I was able to walk all day as a tourist while Paula was at meeting and then go out with her in the evenings. I had not been able to do that for years. At the end of the day the knee ached and I was tired. But, the next day I was able to go again. There were still the issues of having to pay a little more attention to my steps and to going up and down curbs and things. And I was still constantly aware of the joint as I moved around.

Paula could out-walk me for the five years before my surgery. She was now complaining that she was having a hard time keeping up. It was a good feeling to finally be able to out-walk someone. She still insists I may be faster but she can go further. We have not put that theory to the test. I know when to leave well enough alone.

The flight to Chicago was my first airplane experience since the operations. I learned that artificial knees set off metal detectors. I have since learned that a doctor can give the traveler a card saying he or she has prosthetic joint. I never bothered to get a card. All travelers have to go through the metal detector, and once the detector beeps a piece of paper is not going to change what happens after the detector beeps.

My strategy is to go through all the security steps like everyone else. That usually means depositing all metal into your carry-on, removing your shoes, jacket and belt, and piling everything on the conveyor, then standing in front of the metal detector doorway. When the attendant cues me to step through, I announce, "I have artificial knees," step forward and set off the alarm.

I follow the attendant to the individual search area and cooperate while he passes a hand held wand around my body. I visit a little if the attendant is sociable, and tell him where the metal is. The wand goes off at the appropriate joint. The attendant pats me down and sends me on my way. If you are a woman the attendant will be a female.

Living With A Knee Replacement

I was able, with difficulty, to kneel down. Getting down on one knee is a precursor to looking under the bed for a lost shoe, or getting down on the floor to play with grandkids. Kneeling itself at this point is uncomfortable because of the strange sensation on the front of the knee where the nerve has been cut. There is some "feeling" in the area of the knee and putting pressure on it is strange.

Someone once told me that, with a total knee, kneeling would cause the kneecap to shatter. Sometimes the surgery includes hollowing out the back of the knee cap to allow placement of a small plastic button on the backside. My surgeon said the kneecap is quite strong enough to kneel on. The problem with kneeling is simply that it is not very comfortable and I try to avoid the activity. Sitting on a small stool works well for most floor level work. For outside work, such a weeding and transplanting I cut down an old picnic bench to sit on.

There is a way to get to the floor without kneeling at all. Put one foot about a stride forward and bend the knees so your body starts to lower. Put both hands on the floor and move the forward leg back so your legs are together like you were doing a pushup. From that position you can lower one side to the floor and roll onto your bottom. I did this for a while so I could get down and play with my grandkids. As I got stronger it was easier to just kneel down, accepting the odd feelings in the knees, and then sit down on the floor.

With practice, kneeling is not as uncomfortable. At six months post surgery I could kneel for several minutes without any serious problems. I did hear one story, though I could not verify the tale, that a man, ten years after having a knee replaced, laid a hardwood floor. Laying a floor involves a lot of kneeling and I am sure I would not want to try it.

After six months I was brave to put my socks on while standing. Until I was sure of myself, I used the same precautions I had used when learning to put on my pants while standing. I still stand when I put on my socks as a way to make sure I regularly flex the knees as far as they will go. You can also sit down to put your socks on, just remember to pull your knee straight up so it flexes. This trick is another example of how to stretch the knee during normal activities.

I also found the knee had more side to side flexibility. Until about the sixth month when I wanted to turn to one side, I had to stop, lift my feet, and turn each of them in the direction I wanted to go. Now I could swivel my body. The knee itself twisted just fine.

If you are still in the workforce you are probably back at work full time. The healing has progressed enough that you have the energy to do a full day's work, and still have something left over at the end of the day.

PART FOUR:

ENJOY YOUR NEW KNEE

BEYOND SIX MONTHS

The message for this final half-year of healing is that the replacement knee will allow you to get back to your old activities, and maybe try some new things you always wanted to do.

Going into the second half year post surgery the knee feels good. You can have confidence in the new joint. You are ready to venture out and resume a normal life. The key idea is "forget about it." There will be more and more times when you will forget, in the midst of some activity, that you even have a new knee or knees.

FOURTEEN

ALMOST NORMAL: SIX MONTHS AND COUNTING
(This is More What I Was Hoping For)

Now is the time to get back to activities, such as blood donations, charity work, flying, and all the things you might have given up due to the pain before surgery, and could not do during the time it took to recover after the surgery. I had become so physically run down from the pain of limping around on gimpy knees that I let everything else go. I could see that I had not done anything around the house for several years. I had walked as little as possible and was exhausted by the end of the day. I had stopped almost every activity that was not required.

Camping is an important recreation for Paula and me. My inability to walk around the campground with her in the evening was certainly frustrating for her.

After six months I got back to most of those lost activities. I even started to mow the lawn again. It was nice to mow and not be in so much pain I had to rest every fifteen minutes. I started to dig in the garden again. There were still some twinges with a more intense activity like digging, but it was not painful.

Inside activities like cooking and baking became fun again. I love to bake bread and was happy that I could bake without having to hobble around the kitchen.

After the surgery I had taken my bike out to exercise my knee, but did not have the energy to ride to the office, or to the store, or downtown. Now I was taking my bike out for regular rides. The knee was a little stiff at first but loosened up quickly. I had more problems with out of shape muscles that with the knees. That was something I had not expected.

The knee will still let you know that it is there. It pulls and tightens up sat times. However, you can walk on it in confidence, and confidence in the knee is a most important part of recovery. I asked my surgeon what I would be able to do with the artificial knee. He was pretty specific that I could walk on it as much as I wanted. I took him up on it and at the end of a year had worked up to a daily two mile walk. While sightseeing I can walk for hours without pain.

You can overdo it. Gisele told of a day, eight months after her surgery, when she went too far. She was up and about at seven in the morning for a charity event she was working on. During the day she had to go up and down dozens of flights of stairs getting the event set up. Then she walked the three and a half miles of the charity walk. After all that, she gave in to her son's request to ride the paddle boats. She says she suffered for a week.

My doctor also told me that I should not take up furniture moving, weight lifting, shingling, skateboarding or running. My take on that advice is that the knee will hold up well under normal activities but will not take heavy duty demands. My artificial knees are a great excuse to let the young bucks do the heavy lifting.

FIFTEEN

IT ONLY GETS BETTER

Over the second half year the discomfort will continue to lessen. Because the knee is not part of the body's original equipment there may always be some awareness of it. I cannot bend the new knees as far as I could the originals. And it still feels weird when I kneel, though I can get down on my knees when I need to. After a year and a half, I am barely aware of the first knee, a total replacement. I walk two miles a day with my wife, and come home with energy left. I ride my bike, dig in the garden and move an occasional piece of furniture when my wife decides to redecorate. I know many people with prosthetic knees who are golfing, playing tennis, and energetically working full time.

I was surprised at the end of a year when I noticed my balance was back to normal. I had gotten used to watching my steps and being careful to always keep my balance. Then one day I was stepping out of the tub, holding my leg in the air to towel off, when I lost my balance. I realized only later than I had smoothly and easily put my foot down to catch my balance just like I used to do. From that point on I could say I felt normal.

At the end of two years, I find that my knees seem to work even better. Most of the old timers I talk to pay little attention to their new knees. I guess after enough time we can take for granted even what may seem to be a miraculous improvement.

I am now comfortable enough to trust my new knees all the way. My knees are not the way they used to be when I was younger. They are, however, far better than they were before the surgery.

You may wonder how long you can hope to enjoy using your new knee or knees. My surgeon says to look for twenty years of use – more if I'm not too hard on them. Unfortunately, he also said that most knees do not fail because the plastic spacers that stand in for the cartilage wear out. Most prosthetic knees fail because, for some reason, the bond between the appliance and the bone loosens over time. Even so, if the glue lasts for twenty years it has done its job in my book. Over the years the bonding process has improved to almost double the life span of prosthetic knees. But they do not last forever.

During the recovery process I had my leg dropped and fell off steps. I jarred the knee in a near car crash two weeks after surgery and by stubbing my toe. None of these incidents caused any problems other than the original "ouch" response.

I plan to avoid lifting heavy loads that would put additional stress on the bond that holds my wonderful metal and plastic knees in place. I haven't run for twenty-five years, mostly due to having damaged one knee many years ago, and I am not gong to start now. I could run if necessary, but why subject my knees to the pounding that goes with running if there isn't a bear chasing me? When a person is running both feet are off the ground at the same time, so that when each foot hits the ground the full weight of the runner's body comes pounding down on the knee. Elite runners may have a smooth stride that reduces shock, but we weekend joggers do not have that smooth, effortless pace. If you are really into competition race-walking might be an activity your physician would approve. The drawback is that race walkers look like they are waddling along – though at a fast pace.

My plan, at least for the next twenty years, and I'm shooting for thirty, is to actively use my knees walking to sporting events, tourist sites, and lots of other exciting places I used to avoid. I also plan to keep up all those enjoyable activities which put the fun in being alive.

When I went in for my final post-surgery checkup, I told my doctor I was doing fine except for a few twinges. He told me to come back in another year to see if all was well. It's almost that time and I plan to tell him the knees are doing great.

Gisele, my cohort in coming up with the idea for the book emailed a new answer to my question of how often she thinks about her new knee. "One thing I want to share with you is another answer to a question that you asked me which keeps running through my head. You asked me how often I think of my knee. I think about it more often than I realize, but the way I think about it is so different than it was before the surgery. Now when I think of my knee is usually when I'm walking with all my might, keeping up with my son and/or dogs, or hustling to my car because I'm running late (that's all the time). It's a very positive way of thinking in place of a dreadful way of thinking."

On that note I invite you to go out and enjoy your knees.

A brief postscript

It has now been two years since I had the last knee replacement surgery, and the answer to the question of whether Paula or I can walk the furthest has been answered. Recently we went for an evening walk while visiting Omaha. After two hours I was done in – the knees were fine it was just my walking muscles were toast. Paula wanted to go on but graciously agreed to go back to the hotel for my sake. That's love.

Note from Paula: He can ride his bicycle faster and farther than I can, especially uphill! So I guess we each have our strengths! His knee replacements have been a blessing for both of us.

It has been two years now and I find that some of my earlier resolutions have fallen by the wayside. I now will occasionally help Paula move furniture. I dig in the garden without hesitation. I readily kneel when I have to find something on the floor. I do draw the line at crawling around on the floor with the grandkids.

www.ingramcontent.com/pod-product-compliance
Lightning Source LLC
Chambersburg PA
CBHW031211270326
41931CB00006B/513

9 780615 395777